Out *of* Nowhere

Robin Abel and Peggy Sturdivant

LAZY JANE PRODUCTIONS

To the person I love most in the world...my daughter Maria,
Love, Mom

First Edition: May 2010

Lazy Jane Productions

Design and cover illustration by Jo-Ann Sire & John Linse

All photographs unless otherwise attributed are courtesy of Robin Abel's personal photos

Cover art developed from photos admitted as evidence Cause No. 06-02-11563

ISBN 978-0-9845259-0-4

www.outofnowherethebook.com

Printed and bound in Seattle, Washington. United States of America

PART ONE

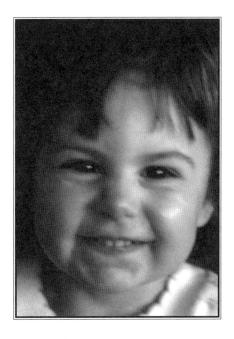

Maria, Age Two

CHAPTER

1

"Dear Ms. Maria Federici,

My husband was driving behind you on the way home from work Sunday night, February 22, 2004. He stopped at the scene of your accident, he broke his way into your vehicle, he heard you breathing, he talked to 9-1-1, he held your hand, he encouraged you to hang in there, . . . he drove home and kissed his three children and wife goodnight. Days later tears still well up in his eyes, for he knows that where his story ends yours begins . . . ."

Note from Mrs. Helene (Anthony) Cox

The movie version of this story could begin with a beautiful, dark-haired woman and her supervisor locking up the bar and restaurant where they work, after a fairly quiet Sunday night. The supervisor, Mason, is fairly new, as is the bartender, Maria. Like most people, he is struck by her beauty, almost distracted by it as they share a steak dinner and a glass of pinot noir for their end-of-shift meal. Maybe he's even a little bit in love with her and would like to believe their employee meal is a date. They walk out to their cars together. There are stars over Lake Washington, and the sky above Seattle is artificially bright. It's not that cold for February. Mason wishes he didn't have to say good night. They get into their cars. For a brief moment he can hear her radio as she turns on the engine. He pulls out of the lot behind her as they both head to the freeway. Mason follows Maria's black Jeep Liberty onto southbound Interstate 405, watching her tail lights ahead of him until he has to exit. Maybe he flashes his headlights or gives a wave as he leaves the freeway. In his head he might be saying, bye, Maria. He might even say it out loud.

But this is where reality takes over. Mason didn't know he would be the last person to look upon the face that had charmed everyone since Maria was born, the first grandchild in her family. And Maria couldn't know that Mason would be the last person she would see before losing her vision. But in the film version, as in real life, the radio is playing, the road is dry, there's very little traffic, until the camera records the deafening crash of breaking glass and crumpling steel. Then all is quiet—except for the radio that continues playing as if nothing has happened.

Robin Abel's life was forever divided into Before and After by the ringing of her rotary phone at around midnight on that February night in 2004. Alone except for her two golden retrievers, she had been asleep in her cabin beside Lake Kathleen.

"Hello," she managed.

A woman's voice said, "I'm calling from Harborview Medical Center."

A pause in the dark.

"Is Maria Federici your daughter?" the woman asked.

For the first time in the twenty-four years she had been Maria's mother, Robin wanted to say, no, she's not my daughter. But already she was saying yes and wondering, oh, Maria, what's happened to you? Robin somehow knew her life was never going to be the same.

"Your daughter's condition is critical," the woman said. "You need to get here as soon as you can. Is there a neighbor who can drive you?"

It seemed so late and dark around the lake.

"Just tell me how to get there," Robin said. The woman explained that Harborview was just three turns from the freeway. Could she get to the freeway?

Hours later, Robin could remember some things but not others. She didn't remember getting dressed or calling her brother's house. All she could think was that she had to get to Harborview but her car was almost out of gas. She felt like screaming as she passed three gas stations, all closed. What was she going to do? What had happened to Maria? At last she saw bright lights at the AM/PM Mini-Mart just before Sunset Highway and the freeway on-ramp.

After filling the tank and getting back in her car, Robin felt sucker-punched, as though she couldn't get a breath. Just breathe, she told herself. She was terrified of driving too fast, having an accident. As she looped onto northbound I-405, she could see the roadway to her left lit by flashing lights and flares, and several emergency vehicles. And then she saw it: a spotlight from one of the aid cars shone directly onto a car, the beam making the cracked windshield glass sparkle. It looked like Maria's Jeep Liberty.

Jean Gamboa had driven the exact route between work and home for years, five nights a week. The route took her from the Albertson's Grocery Store on Mercer Island to her house in Covington. As a divorced single parent, she was particularly careful not to take risks. Her number one rule was that she never, ever stopped on the roads at night.

On the night of Maria's accident, Jean's shift had ended at ten o'clock. The roads were dry. There wasn't much traffic on I-405. She was in a very familiar groove, radio on. She was in the right-hand lane, driving exactly the speed limit in her Dodge Caravan.

A vehicle ahead of her, a black SUV, moved into her lane

and became a pair of tail lights well in front. Then something happened. A sudden storm of debris sent pieces of wood flying up from the vehicle. Several pieces hit Jean's car. The SUV slowed gradually and drifted to a stop against the shoulder barrier. Jean hit her flashers as she followed the vehicle to the shoulder, her wheels continuing to hit debris. The SUV was smoking. Believing that the driver of the car was a woman, Jean wondered if she was okay. Then she did something she had never done in all of her years of commuting at night. She got out of her car and walked toward the unknown.

That night, Anthony Cox was also on his way home from work on I-405. He was a bus driver for King County Metro, a job he'd held for nearly thirty years. Trained to be alert to potential hazards, even on a night with clear roads and very few other vehicles, Anthony took note of the black Jeep to the right of him, moving at about the same speed as he was. Suddenly, he saw debris bouncing off the Jeep and sparks coming from its undercarriage. He watched as the Jeep slowed and then stopped on the shoulder, its hood up. Something was terribly wrong, he thought. Anthony decided to pull over and see if he could help, parking well in front of the Jeep and another car that had pulled in behind it. As he ran back to the Jeep, he noticed that another person was approaching the vehicle on foot.

Jean and Anthony didn't introduce themselves as they tried to open the driver's side door of the Jeep, yet they were paired in an instant. The door was locked, but through the window they could see the driver slumped over onto the passenger side. The windshield was shattered.

"There's a blanket in my car," Anthony yelled. "Get it."

Jean ran toward his car but it seemed so far away. By the time she returned with the blanket, Anthony had climbed on top of the hood, broken through the windshield, and reached through the glass to unlock the door from the inside. The keys were in the ignition and the radio was still playing. Jean handed him the blanket through the open car door, and he wrapped it over the driver's body, now curled into a fetal position. A large board jutted through the windshield and onto the steering wheel. Jean could see blood illuminated by the dome light.

"Do you have a phone?" Anthony asked. "Call 9-1-1"

A woman's voice answered and Jean tried to speak. "There's been an accident. We're on 405."

"Northbound or southbound?" the dispatcher asked her. "Do you know your location?"

Jean wasn't sure anymore. She could see an exit sign on the northbound side. "It's near an overpass," she said. "I can't see the exit number. It's near Sunset. There are lights."

Then she couldn't go on speaking–or even standing. She managed to hand the phone to Anthony, who was leaning into the front of the car, feeling for a pulse on the woman slumped on the seat. Jean slid down the side of the car. She could hear him talking on the phone and to the woman in the Jeep. She sat watching for emergency lights. Why did it take so long? Why didn't anyone else stop? How could other cars keep driving by?

Anthony leaned closer to the driver's head. He heard her making a noise, a gurgling sound as though she were choking.

"Hang in there," he said to her, holding her hand. "We're getting you help." He knew there was a lot of blood because he could feel its sticky heat on his hand, even though her hand was cold. He couldn't make out any features of her face. He leaned closer to see if she was still breathing. Anthony could smell the woman's hair shampoo.

Jean managed to stand up when two emergency vehicles arrived, a fire engine and a smaller aid truck. They stopped in the right-hand lane of traffic and two men strode toward her. One looked like a giant.

"We'll take over," one man said to Anthony. They reached in and tossed out the blanket. Then it seemed to Jean that they reached in and just pulled out the young woman. Other firemen were putting out cones and flares to block the lanes of traffic. Jean had the impression of more flashing lights arriving and firemen asking her if she was all right. Emergency workers eased the woman onto a stretcher and put her into the back of an ambulance. It pulled out onto the freeway almost immediately, leaving Jean, Anthony, and so many flashing lights.

"Come sit down in here for a bit," a fireman said, leading Jean to an aid truck. She sat inside next to Anthony, whose hands were covered by glass and blood from breaking the windshield. He kept rubbing them, trying to clear the glass.

"Don't rub them," the fireman said. "Let's try to clean them out. What are your names?"

Jean and Anthony looked at each other as though they should already know. They said their names for the fireman. Alone together for fifteen minutes, they had been a team, trying to help the injured woman. A fireman took Jean's pulse and looked into her eyes with a penlight.

"I can't stop shaking," she told him.

"You're still in a slight state of shock," he told her. "It will pass."

They poured water over Anthony's hands, then looked to see if there was more glass. The engine of the ambulance was running, and Jean felt as though she were breathing pure exhaust. So she went outside, where a sheriff or State Patrol person asked her to fill out paperwork.

"We need a report from you before you leave," an officer said. They gave her a form and a pen. Jean just looked at it. She couldn't have gone anywhere even if she had felt capable of driving; her car was blocked in and two lanes of the freeway were still closed. It seemed strange to her that two lanes had been closed for an accident where only two people had even stopped.

"Have you finished your report?" the sheriff asked her. Jean couldn't write. She couldn't even stop shaking. She called out to a firefighter. "The woman who was injured, is she going to be okay?" She remembers that he said, "No."

Jean went to her car and tried to do the report. She couldn't fix her eyes on the paper. An officer tapped at the window. "Do you have the report?" he asked.

"I can't do this now," she said.

Nobody asked if there was anyone she could call. No one asked if she was all right to drive home. Anthony, evidently, had already done his report and left. His car had been in front of the emergency vehicles. Jean was the only remaining witness. An officer said she could take the report with her, but she needed to give them her name and phone number and a few facts about what had happened. Jean made another attempt to fill out the form, then asked the officer again.

"The woman who was in the Jeep, is she going to be okay?"

Again she was told, "No." Jean sat a few more minutes and then managed to turn the ignition key and start her car. She wondered if she should ask a third person about the woman's condition. It seemed like she should keep asking until somebody told her, "Yes." She didn't think she could stand it if the woman didn't survive.

She drove home, her hands tingling on the steering wheel. When she got there she went in and made sure her daughter was sleeping. She crawled into her bed but couldn't fall asleep. With her eyes closed, she could still see debris hitting the car, the flashing lights of the emergency vehicles, the young woman lying on the pavement.

When she reached Harborview Hospital, Robin pulled her Volkswagen Beetle into a parking space outside the entrance marked "Emergency." She wondered if it would all right to park there. What if I get a ticket? she thought. Then she realized how crazy it was to worry about something like that when she didn't even know what had happened to Maria. She wanted to believe she was wrong about seeing an accident on the freeway involving a car identical to Maria's.

Robin had never been to Harborview before, although she had heard about it for years in the news. She pushed through the doors and stopped at the entrance to the waiting room. It was filled with people, but strangely quiet. There was no one at the reception desk. Her head was filled with questions. If someone didn't appear, she felt as if she would scream. Then she saw someone who looked like she worked there.

"You called about my daughter, Maria Federici," Robin said.

"Hold on," the woman said, and a few moments later someone came out and introduced herself as a social worker.

"I'm Maria's mom," Robin told her.

"Let's find someplace more private," the social worker said, leading Robin to a closed door.

As the social worker put her hand on the doorknob, Robin grabbed her forearm. "Is my daughter still alive?" she asked.

The social worker replied, "I don't know."

CHAPTER

2

"Twenty-four-year-old female, chief complaint is face struck by plywood while driving southbound on I-405. Wood came through the windshield and struck her horizontally in the face, devastating her eyes, nose, and upper mandible. She was rapidly extricated and aggressively bagged with a bag valve mask by Renton Fire Department. Medic One called."

Harborview Medical Center Emergency Department notes

Jim Stevens was on call with Medic One on the day of Maria's accident. He and his partner, Steve Perry, were at the Renton station, south of Seattle, when they got the call. Medic One is the elite of medical response; the program, started through Harborview, has become an international model for reducing mortality in the field. Medic One responders are specially trained to begin life-saving procedures that would otherwise not be possible outside of an emergency room. On their way to the scene Stevens and Perry received a short report from the first responders, who called the situation "fairly grim." Aid Unit 12 reported that a woman had been driving her car when a board came through the windshield and hit her in the face. Stevens and his partner tried to anticipate how to treat that type of injury, but they really didn't know what to expect.

The Medic One paramedics pulled up behind the Renton aid truck on southbound I-405. Perry stayed in the truck to prepare an intubation kit and intravenous fluids. Stevens got out the gurney and pushed it toward the victim. "Let's get her in the truck," he called out to the emergency medical technicians working on Maria.

The Engine 12 lieutenant stepped toward him. "You might want to take a peek before you do anything else," he said.

The lieutenant was highly experienced, and Stevens knew he was implying that the victim might have already expired. Approaching the spot where the EMTs were working on Maria, Stevens recognized two people he knew from several years working in the south end, Doug and Orson. One EMT was doing chest compressions while the other was trying to help the woman breathe.

Doug looked up and said, "I don't think I'm doing her any good with this bag valve mask."

They straightened up so that Stevens could have a look. No one who saw the damage to the young woman has ever been able to forget the sight, but what Stevens registered first was that she was still trying to breathe.

"Let's get her in the truck," Stevens said again. "We can put a tube in to help her get some air."

With one person holding her head and two others supporting her body, they log rolled her onto a carrying board. The facial injuries were obvious, but they had to assume there might also be spinal or internal injuries. As they placed the carrying board on the gurney, Stevens could see that the woman had a horrific facial injury, the most severe he had ever encountered.

They secured the gurney inside the Medic One truck and drove off immediately. One of the EMTs from Aid 12 rode in the back with them and another EMT took the wheel for the drive to Harborview. Steve Perry managed to get a tracheal breathing tube through the vocal cords. Stevens attempted to insert tubing at a standard site to be able to deliver fluids, but then moved to a subclavian intravenous, just below the collar bone. He began giving Maria a saline solution known as lactated ringers, because she had obviously lost a lot of blood before they had arrived, and was still losing it. Her pulse was very faint, her blood pressure extremely low.

It was Stevens' job to try to keep Maria alive until they reached Harborview, monitoring her vital signs and logging any procedures they performed. He couldn't quantify how much blood she had lost. He could only track the fluids they administered. In the twelve minutes it took them to reach Harborview, he and his partner gave her 2.7 liters of fluid, almost half the amount in the average human body.

Stevens and Perry were following the A-B-C life-saving protocol–Airway-Breathing-Circulation–in that order. Victims can't survive if their airways are obstructed. Oxygen needs to get in and carbon dioxide needs to get out. The medics had inserted a breathing tube, known as a "cuffed tracheal," which inflates and seals off the airway to protect the lungs from other fluids, such as blood or vomit. The cuffed tracheal tube is considered the gold standard for protecting the airway in an injury.

With the cuffed tracheal tube in place, Maria's blood oxygen had come up slightly. Next was the circulatory system. Places in the body that are inclined to blush, the head and neck particularly, are full of blood vessels and prone to bleeding. Given that her injuries were craniofacial, the blood loss was so profound that Stevens and Perry knew Maria was at risk of bleeding out completely.

They wrapped her face in a special type of gauze called Kerlix. It took them four rolls. Though they were not attempting to pack her wounds, the effect was similar because of its absorbency. Then they were able to proceed with assessing her condition before transferring Maria to the trauma doctor waiting for them at Harborview.

Under "severity of the injury," they marked the box for "life-threatening." On the scale used to rate injuries, Maria's score was close to most dire: four on a scale of three to fifteen. Her carbon dioxide output was nine, with thirty-two considered normal. At one point on the way to Harborview, her blood pressure went below sixty, so they did chest compressions. She was unconscious and non-responsive.

They had radioed Harborview to prepare for the arrival of a life-threatening injury. Their rig came to a stop in the ambulance bay. Stevens and Perry slid the gurney out and hurried to Recess Two in the emergency department. Stevens briefed the attending doctor on Maria's vitals and what they had done en route. Their contact with the patient was now finished. All that remained was writing up the paperwork and cleaning their rig to be ready for the next call.

In almost ten years as a medic and paramedic, Stevens had not seen a person survive an injury as bad as Maria's. On the way back to the station Stevens thought about a video he'd seen during Medic One training. It documented an incident where a man had tried to commit suicide with a shotgun. It was particularly gruesome because the man nearly carved a canoe vertically through his face. But he had survived. Stevens thought to himself, if that man survived something that he did to himself, maybe this young woman can live through something that wasn't her fault.

Stevens didn't learn until later that within the next hour the trauma team at Harborview deemed her injuries "incompatible with life."

Robin, after arriving at Harborview, was placed in what she later learned was called a "quiet room." A social worker sat with her, but Robin doesn't recall talking to her. What she remembers best is when a door opened and two doctors entered and stood over her. She looked up at them, trying to read their faces. Why didn't they say anything, she wondered? Their coats were so clean, so white. There was no blood. Surely everything was all right.

"Can you save her?" Robin asked them.

They shook their heads.

This can't be happening, Robin thought. They haven't even told me what happened to my daughter.

"Are you sure you can't save her?" she asked again.

The two doctors then told Robin that Maria had been brought to the emergency room by Medic One in severe trauma, with injuries to multiple systems. She had major facial injuries, but the worst of the damage was that she was bleeding out from the center of her brain. "Bleeding out" is different than just blood loss. They said they'd tried for almost an hour, but they couldn't stop the bleeding. Maria had a pulse and was breathing with assistance, they said, but still "it was just a matter of time." They left the words 'before she died' unsaid but they hung in the air.

Robin sat in shock. Throughout her life, Robin had always tried to rescue every creature she encountered, from injured rabbits and birds to dogs with broken backs. Her daughter thought she could heal any animal. The doctors stood silent, as if waiting for a response. It occurred to Robin that they were there for another reason.

"Are you here for her organs?" she whispered.

They nodded yes. Of course, Robin thought, Maria would want to save other people's lives. Robin felt that if her daughter's organs could spare another family from hearing that their child or loved one didn't have a chance, she would give permission to the doctors.

"She would want that," Robin told them.

The social worker asked, "Are there any family members you can call?"

15

"Bobby's on his way," she said, "My brother." It was the only thing that made any sense at that moment. This might be a mistake. Bobby would sort it out.

When Maria was clocked into the emergency room at Harborview, Dr. John Westhoff was the senior resident in charge of surgical services on that shift. In his role as trauma doctor, his job was to direct the arriving patient's care, under the supervision of the chief resident of general surgery. Westhoff had served a year as Chief of the Emergency Department for the 21st Combat Support Hospital in Baghdad, treating everything that came through the door. But nothing had prepared him for Maria's injuries. The Medic One unit had told Harborview dispatch that Maria's injury was "devastating," and recommended that general surgical services be called. So Westhoff was standing by when Maria was rolled into the hospital.

As he unraveled the rolls of Kerlix that covered her face, he was relieved to see that her airway had been secured; otherwise she would not have survived transport. Then he started examining her wounds. He knew he was looking at a face, but there was not a single recognizable feature all the way down to her chin. Beneath her obliterated eye sockets there was only a concavity filled with blood and tissue. She was bleeding from her face in a constant steady stream. Westhoff and his team started a second intravenous line to introduce additional blood products, packed red cells, plasma, platelets, and more saline. Westhoff could see from the Medic One notes and the ongoing blood loss that she was acidotic, meaning that her blood pH was completely off; her tissues weren't getting oxygenated blood. He knew that this could cause tissue and organ death.

Her bleeding was like a broken dam; it was no use pumping her with blood when it was flowing out faster than they could get it into her. Westhoff tried to figure out how to stop the bleeding. He packed her face but it didn't help. "We need to stop this bleeding," he told the chief resident, who responded that they first needed to know the cause and extent of the blood loss. After ordering computerized tomography, better known as CT scan, the chief resident left to attend to other duties.

Westhoff tried to do the CT, which usually provides an accurate view of soft tissues. But Maria's blood was pouring onto the machine, preventing it from working. He sent his junior residents to find the chief resident again.

"Tell him that he's got to come back here now!" he said.

When the chief resident returned, Westhoff told him, "We've got to do something because I can't keep up. I can't keep giving her blood as fast as she is losing blood."

All the residents could see that ordinary procedures no long applied. Maria was bleeding out quickly and they couldn't tell why. The chief resident decided to send for the chief neurosurgery resident. There wasn't even time to move her to an operating room, so they began to operate right there in the emergency department, in a desperate effort to stop Maria from losing all of the blood in her body.

Thanks to the tracheal tube, her lungs were still working. And her heart was still trying to pump blood to her brain. But most of that blood was ending up on the floor, on the gurney, on the CT machine. Vital oxygen wasn't getting delivered to her brain, and carbon dioxide wasn't getting removed. It appeared that Maria's carotid arteries–blood vessels that provide blood directly from the heart to the brain–had probably been severed just at the point where they enter the brain. When the surgeons clamped the vessels, her bleeding slowed and then mostly stopped.

The bleeding crisis was over, but lying on the gurney was a young woman who had lost the blood supply to her brain. All three surgeons standing beside Maria thought that her injuries were incompatible with life.

"Non-survivable injury," a resident wrote on her chart.

Someone in the room said, "Better contact LifeCenter

Northwest," referring to the local organ donation organization. The surgeons saw viable organs in an otherwise healthy young woman–as long as she was kept alive through life support. Maria was an excellent candidate for organ donation, but Westhoff first needed to talk to the mother.

Robin remembers multiple doctors in coats that were too white. But Westhoff remembers he was alone with her. The other surgeons weren't available for the first contact, and he was the attending that night. He told Robin that other surgeons would be in to talk to her about the specifics of her daughter's injury, but that it was very, very serious. He didn't mention organ donation at that point, although he was privy to the plan to notify LifeCenter Northwest. Especially when a patient is still technically alive, doctors try to prepare the family for the prognosis, careful not to convey false hope. Maria would still need to be carefully assessed for brain function, but Westhoff was setting the stage for the statistical unlikelihood that she would survive. He wouldn't deliver the bad news until later.

During the course of her surgery, surgeons had transfused Maria with twelve units of packed red blood cells, a concentrate of the most essential part of the blood. In addition, she'd been given seven liters of plasma and two liters of lactated ringers, or saline solution, plus the 2.7 liters of fluids administered by Medic One. It was an astonishing amount of fluids and blood products for such a small woman.

Westhoff wrote the orders for Maria to be transferred from the emergency department to the surgical intensive care unit, or ICU, along with instructions to administer fluids that would keep her organs viable. The neurosurgeon had noted that she was not responding to painful stimuli nor making any spontaneous movement. It was likely that she was brain dead. He wrote the words "comfort care" on her chart. The last four words were the bottom line: "Hold for LifeCenter NW."

With that, Maria left Westhoff's care. As per standing orders, the Director of Emergency Services, Dr. Michael Copass, was informed that a patient from Medic One had been admitted to the ICU and was not expected to survive till morning.

Maria's injuries had been dramatic even by the standards of a Level One trauma center, a hospital designed to handle the most life-threatening injuries. When Westhoff returned to work the following night, he inquired about Maria because he had not been able to get her case out of his mind.

CHAPTER

3

On the night of Maria's accident, as Robin made her way to Harborview, she called her brother's home. Her sister-in-law, Kim, answered the phone.

"Robin?" Kim said. "What's wrong?"

Bobby heard his wife say, "Maria" and "how serious?" He was out of bed and starting to put his clothes on as Kim, keeping Robin on the line, told him the news.

"Maria's been in an accident," she said "You need to meet Robin at Harborview."

Robin was the oldest of Bobby's three sisters. His wife kept talking to Robin while she followed him out to their car. They lived across Puget Sound from Seattle. At that hour of the morning, the ferries didn't operate, so he would have to drive across the Narrows Bridge and north through Tacoma.

"You need to breathe," he heard Kim tell Robin. "You can do this."

Bobby pulled out of the driveway and began the series of turns that led to the highway. He knew the route to Seattle well, could time it almost to the minute on such a clear Sunday night. Seventy minutes on a night without traffic. It was just after 1:00 a.m.

As he drove, Bobby called Robin on his wife's cell phone, which was actually the official town phone of Port Orchard where his wife was mayor. Robin was still en route to Harborview. While they were talking, Robin spotted what she thought was Maria's Jeep on the southbound side just as she got on the freeway

Bobby found his way to Harborview's Emergency Room entrance. He felt stupid and helpless as he waited for someone to assist him. Then he was led to where Robin was sitting alone in a small windowless room. His sister's skin looked grey, even her voice seemed leaden.

"Bobby," Robin said. "They say Maria's gone."

Robin's family, including her grandparents, had lived in Seattle her entire life. She grew up in West Seattle, the oldest of Bob and JoRene Abel's four children. There was Robin, Susan, Bobby, and Lizzie, the baby. Even when Bobby had grown taller than his dad, he remained Little Bob to her dad's Big Bob. They lived just blocks from Lincoln Park and the Fauntleroy ferry dock. They all loved animals and playing in the water.

In the summer they'd go to their cabin, nicknamed The Lazy Jane, on Lake Kathleen, in the town of Renton, south of Seattle. Robin and Susan had horses. Bobby had a pony. They all slept outdoors and rowed and fished. They swam and played horseshoes, often competing in tournaments with each other and all the other children camped nearby. There were always neighborhood picnics.

Robin considered herself a tomboy, even during the stage when she wanted to be a professional gymnast. She was independent, too, working from a young age, saving her money to buy property. Her marriage and pregnancy were a shock at first, especially as the pregnancy had come before the marriage. She was building a log cabin on Whidbey Island through her whole pregnancy. Maria Christina Federici was born on Halloween when Robin was twenty-five years old. Federici was the father's surname. It was important to Robin that Maria wasn't considered illegitimate by the definitions of the Coupeville hospital, so she gave her daughter her father's name. But within a year, Robin and Maria were on their own–by choice.

Maria was the first grandchild and beautiful from the day she gave her first toothless smile. Robin's sister, Susan, and her husband, Richard, had a little girl, Kristina, a year later. Maria and Kristina were like sisters for many years, spending time together with their grandparents. They were smart, precious girls who were spoiled and adored by the whole Abel clan. Maria was always the more dramatic of the two, striking a pose in every photo.

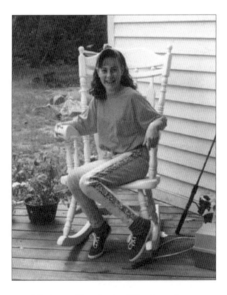

Maria on the deck of the Lazy Jane

All through grade school and high school Maria always had good grades and seemed to make friends effortlessly. She would bake cookies for the neighbors, delivering them in the company of her dog, Arthur, a German pointer. Artie, she called him. When she was eight years old Robin had decided to fix up the family cabin on the lake to live in year-round. At first Maria swore she wouldn't live there, but when she got back from a summer visit with her dad she was impressed with her mother's remodeling work. "It's rad," she said, giving her mother the thumbs up.

Maria never had a gawky stage. Not even braces detracted from the huge brown eyes and warm smile. By her early twenties she was glamorously beautiful. Maria had the figure, the eyes, the hair, the voice, but some people didn't realize how smart she was beneath those looks. Everybody liked Maria; even ex-boyfriends became friends. She was one of those people everyone wanted to be near, as though her vivaciousness were transferable.

It seemed like her accomplishments came easily to her, but she always worked hard. She earned a partial scholarship at the University of Washington; her father paid the other half. Maria worked two or three jobs all through college to pay for her living expenses and to buy her books. Robin let her live at home while she went to the University; she had moved out about a year before the accident.

After Bobby found his sister at Harborview, she explained to him that the doctors gave Maria little hope of survival. They had told her that both of Maria's carotid arteries had been severed. They'd used the term "facial avulsion," and when Robin just stared up at them blankly, one of the doctors translated for her: Maria's face and the frontal lobe of her brain had been destroyed. She told Bobby that she had not yet seen her daughter.

"I don't want to see Maria without a face," she said to Bobby.

Bobby Abel is a scientist. But he's also a man who grew up with three sisters. In his work and teaching he deals with data, measurements, predictable outcomes. He believes in doing what needs to be done. Digging fence posts, bicycling in any weather, never siding with one sister over another, plugging away at a problem over and over until he can unlock the solution like a riddle. He knew that his older sister needed him to be her witness to Maria, to see if it was true what had happened, because how could it be that her daughter had "nonsurvivable injuries?"

"I'll go see her," Bobby said.

A nurse took him to what appeared to be a small operating room. Next to the covered body on a gurney were poles hung with bags of fluid, one clear, one dark red. A towel covered the area where her face should have been. Emerging from the towel was a white plastic tube attached to an oxygen system. He saw a hint of Maria's dark hair at the edge of the towel, next to gauze soaked with blood. Bob reached for her hand, looking to the nurse for guidance. The nurse nodded his approval. Bob held her hand. It was all he could do. Blood was running down her arm. He watched helplessly as it dripped and splashed on his shoes. He thought about how he would have to wipe his shoes so Robin wouldn't see the blood.

As a person who needs facts, Bob began asking questions about Maria's status. The nurse made notes in a chart, recording data from the monitors, then retrieved notes from the emergency technicians at the scene. He told Bob what they had said: an object had gone through her Jeep's windshield and through her face. They had managed to protect an airway in the field, and she had arrived at Harborview within thirty minutes of the 9-1-1 call.

"What happens now?" Bob asked.

"LifeCenter Northwest has been called," the nurse told him, referring to the potential organ donation. "We keep her as comfortable as possible. But you'll need to speak with her doctors."

Bob tried to clean the blood from his shoes with paper towels. By the time he returned to Robin, other members of the family had arrived in response to his wife's phone calls. His two other sisters were there. Even his sister's ex-husband, Richard, had come with his daughter Kristina.

As Robin's family continued to arrive, Harborview workers shifted them to various rooms tucked into the basement. A woman arrived from LifeCenter NW and took Robin and Bobby to a conference room to work on forms. Robin began to cry. The questions were very personal, asking for a full medical history to date, and about drug and alcohol use. These questions would have seemed too private in the best of circumstances but now just seemed painful. It came down to signing forms that agreed to donate any viable organs.

Robin turned to Bobby, pen poised.

"But she's still alive," Robin said. "There might be hope."

Her brother shook his head and met her eyes. "Robin, she's dead. Sign the papers."

Robin wiped away tears so that she could see to sign, then pushed away all the forms.

"I need to say goodbye," she said. "But I can't bear to remember her without a face."

"They'll take care of it," Bobby said. He went to find a nurse or doctor.

For Robin's farewell to her daughter, Maria's nurse placed a fresh towel over her face. Robin approached her daughter, afraid of what she would see. Above the towel her finely shaped eyebrows were still intact. In fact Maria looked surprisingly normal from the top of her eyebrows up through her hairline. Clearly this couldn't be that bad, Robin thought. She reached out to hold her hand. It was cold and felt grossly swollen. Then something odd happened. Robin felt Maria's hand move a little.

"She moved!" Robin told the nurse. "Her hand moved."

The nurse responded that it was an involuntary movement, not a sign of brain activity.

"Are you sure?" Robin asked. It was true that Maria was very still. She was almost never this still, even in her sleep.

The nurse nodded yes.

The moment seemed completely unreal to Robin. She felt almost numb.

"I love you so much, Maria," Robin said to her. "I'm so proud of you but I need to say goodbye."

She stood beside Maria, somehow certain that if she waited long enough Maria would respond. Bobby put his arm around her shoulders and walked her away from her daughter.

It was not quite dawn when the Abel family walked out of Harborview together. It had been decided that Bobby would drive Robin, in her car, back to the cabin to pick up her dogs and take all of them to his house in Port Orchard. Bobby's concern was taking care of Robin and getting her home to his wife. Although she happened to be Mayor of Port Orchard no one could be more comforting than Kim.

He drove but doesn't remember the route, other than avoiding southbound Interstate 405. They must have taken I-5 instead. Robin was crying and talking about times when Maria was a child, always listening for her footsteps on the deck when she was outside. Maria would come in and say, "I'm home, Mom."

Then Robin asked Bobby abruptly, "What happened? Do you know what happened to her?"

Bobby told her what the nurse had told him. A large board had flown through her windshield and struck her directly in the face. Other drivers had stopped and called 9-1-1. They didn't have more details.

"I saw her car," Robin said. "I saw her car on 405. The windshield was broken where her face should have been."

"I know," he told her. "You were talking to me when you saw it."

"I was?" Robin said. She couldn't remember anything but the sight of the emergency vehicles and spotlight on the windshield.

"Oh, God," she said suddenly. "Where will I bury her?"

Bobby let her keep talking. It was as though she was just speaking her thoughts out loud as they came to her.

"There's the cemetery near the cabin," she said. "Where Jimi Hendrix is buried. Maria would appreciate that."

Bobby had never been in a situation like this before. For all their antics at the lake and horseback riding, no one in the family had ever been seriously hurt. They'd escaped broken bones and concussions, car accidents and heart attacks. Robin was the sister who had always protected him. She'd rescued his GI Joe when it went out too deep in the water. She'd watched out for him as the only girl on the neighborhood softball team. She had always been there for him.

He was trained in physics, not social work. How the hell was he going to be able to help Robin? At the hospital, he had tried to help her complete the social and medical history for the organ donation questionnaire. He'd taken the bereavement kit from the social worker for Robin. He'd been so worried that Robin would see all the blood on Maria; thank goodness they had cleaned her up before Robin went in to say goodbye.

Bobby took the Sunset exit that would lead them back to Robin's cabin. The lights went on inside an espresso drive-up shaped like a mini-caboose. He looked at Robin and she nodded. After ordering, they realized that neither was carrying any money, until Robin looked down at Maria's purse in her lap. They'd given it to Robin at the hospital. She dug out the wallet, tears running down her face. "This one's on Maria," Robin said, and gestured to Bobby to put the change from a twenty-dollar bill directly into the tip jar.

"Maria made her living from tips," Robin said. "She'd want us to tip really well this morning."

As soon as Robin and Bobby went inside the cabin, both wanted to leave as quickly as possible. It was dangerous with memories. They loaded her two golden retrievers, Beau and Jorja, and dog food into Robin's Volkswagen. Robin kept talking about Maria, how she had rarely been sick, only needing to have her tonsils removed, how she had always been so healthy. Bobby concentrated on driving them back around the land route to Port Orchard, seventy minutes on a good day. The irony of the phrase struck him: this had been anything but a good day.

Bobby had called Kim throughout the night and then again when he had left Harborview to drive Robin to the cabin. "Your parents are on their way," Kim told him. They would be on the first flight from Las Vegas and then join them in Port Orchard. Kim had sent the boys off to school, so she was alone when she heard Robin's car in the driveway. Kim went outside to meet them.

Kim had held Maria on the day she was born. When Kim and Bobby were married two years later, in West Seattle's Lincoln Park, Maria was there with her knees still toddler-chubby. All big dark eyes and dark hair, Maria stood out in a family that ran to blonds and redheads; she was the only one with her grandmother JoRene's coloring. As the years went by, other nephews and nieces were born, on both her side of the family and on Bobby's, and then their own two boys, Kellen and Riley. The boys were much younger than their cousins, who loved to give them gifts and dress them up like little Ken dolls.

Kim didn't love shopping for clothes as much as Bobby's sisters did; she didn't have what was laughingly referred to as the "shopping gene." Instead of giving Maria clothes, Kim used to read with her, as she was an early reader who loved books.

One of Kim's favorite memories of Maria as a child was when the little girl would accompany her mother on weekend real estate appraisals. "What are you doing today?" Kim would ask Maria.

" 'Spections and 'praisals,'" Maria always said.

Inside the house Kim and Robin sat on the couch and just cried together. Bob took a shower and left on his bicycle for Olympia College to teach his classes. Later on, they would all wonder why he did that. But nothing made sense to him other than pretending their world hadn't been devastated. It didn't occur to Bob to try to cancel or find a substitute until it was too late.

Robin and Kim talked more about Maria, tears coming often. Then, when they had reached a brief cried-out stage, Robin's phone rang. Kim answered it for her. It was someone from Harborview, so she passed the phone to Robin. On morning rounds, doctors had noticed that Maria seemed to be experiencing pain, which meant she was no longer unresponsive. Maria still had a chance, Robin and Kim both thought. In that moment, Kim felt it go from darkest night to dawn, as though their hearts had been flat-lined but suddenly returned to a rhythm.

"I have to go back," Robin said.

Perhaps because Robin's dad's family had moved around so much, Big Bob and his wife, JoRene, settled in West Seattle once they had children, and stayed there until he retired. Bob had served in the Navy and had graduated from the University of Washington when he caught a glimpse of a beautiful girl, who lived a few doors away from where he was working on the family house in the South Park area of Seattle. Family lore has it that Bob fell off the roof when he first spotted JoRene.

Unlike Bob, JoRene had lived her entire life in just one home in South Park. She'd even been crowned Queen of South Park. Bob was in law school when they first started dating. They got married in Madison Park, near Lake Washington, on November 18, 1949. Today, nearly sixty years later, they are still just as smitten.

Robin was their first-born, red-faced and white-blonde. Of their four children—two girls, a son, and then another daughter—Robin was the one who always had to be with her dad. When he was building their home in West Seattle, she was loading the wheelbarrow. If he was going fishing, she was going with him, and she was the only one of his children who seemed to need fishing like other people need books or music. Robin even followed her dad into the banking profession.

It was a magical time in Seattle as the Abel children grew up. Living near the Fauntleroy ferry dock by Lincoln Park, in West Seattle, their house was always filled with animals. The kids once tried to smuggle an abandoned kitten back from Lake Fenwick, covering the meows by singing loudly the entire way home, in a revealing display of unity. "Shall we stop at the store to pick up cat food?" their dad asked.

The family bought a lamb to keep the blackberry bushes in check, and Robin would take it for walks on a leash. A policeman stopped her once just to satisfy his curiosity. "It is a lamb," he said.

In the summer, the Abel family went to their cabin at Lake Kathleen. JoRene's best friend would stay next door with her four children, along with her sisters and all of their children. It was like a sleep-away camp with all the kids in sleeping bags outside in the cabana, horses to ride, row boats to take out to the lake. They held their own mini-Olympics, setting up events and awarding medals. There were no fences between the cabins then, and the children all played as one huge, extended family. The towheads were the Abel kids: Robin, Susan, Bobby, and Liz.

Then there was Sam Dog–a sheep dog who followed the Abel kids home during a snowstorm. Even though his owner claimed him, the dog always returned to the Abel home; the dog would be at the back door, his owner at the front. For several months there was a custody battle of sorts, with the dog's owner threatening to sue for breach of affection. Eventually the owner gave up trying to take Sam home and he became the Abel's dog. The dog lived so long that he attended Bobby's wedding to Kim in Lincoln Park.

JoRene met each of her grandchildren right after he or she was born, starting with Maria on Whidbey Island. JoRene knew just how to wrap the babies in their receiving blankets, rolling in one side, pulling up the bottom, and then tightly wrapping the other side into the perfect burrito. Babies need to be tightly wrapped when they are newly born, JoRene believed, so that their own limbs don't scare them. She wrapped all six of her grandchildren like that so they would know they were safe.

When Kim phoned JoRene on the night of Maria's accident, JoRene had already made a reservation to fly from Las Vegas to Seattle later in the week. They still had a cabin in Gig Harbor and had been going back and forth for years now, JoRene more frequently than Bob, who had been diagnosed with Parkinson's disease. Kim told her that Maria had been seriously injured and might not survive. Kim admitted that Robin had already been asked about organ donation.

JoRene did not allow herself to think beyond the need to get both Bob and herself to Seattle as quickly as possible, on the first flight of the day. Five hundred miles per hour is not fast enough for a mother who needs to get to her children and grandchildren.

Just before they boarded the plane, JoRene talked to Bobby at the hospital. He told her, "Mom, Robin has signed the papers. They've told us to say our goodbyes."

Two hours later, as the plane pulled up to its gate in Seattle, an announcement came over the intercom, "Would Mr. and Mrs. Robert Abel please identify themselves to a flight attendant?" JoRene raised her hand. Within moments, her daughter, Susan, who worked at the airport, was hustling down the aisle to get them off the plane first. Susan had pulled strings to have their luggage unloaded immediately and a car waiting.

As Robin's parents pulled into Bobby and Kim's driveway, Robin came out of the house to meet them. "Maria's still alive," she said. "We're going back to the hospital."

Chief Investigating Detective Nathan Elias of the Washington State Patrol was older than he looked. Despite his teenage looks, he had done years of accident investigation for what is the largest public safety law enforcement agency in the state of Washington. The first trooper at the scene began a report and called for the investigation team. Elias led the troopers as they gathered evidence almost continually for twelve hours. He would revisit the scene many times over the next weeks, and return to it mentally for years.

It was remarkable to Elias that Maria's black Jeep Liberty had come to rest against the barrier at the side of the roadway, almost like a Puget Sound ferry scraping gently into a pier. Yet a black, six-foot by two-foot sheet of particle board had hit the driver and was still lying on the steering wheel. Despite what he had witnessed over the years, Elias was sometimes forced to believe in sheer good luck. Certainly the driver was not lucky to be at the exact time and place a huge object of unknown origin flew in her path. But she was lucky that she had not ricocheted into another vehicle or even flipped into the northbound lanes.

The debris path stretched for almost 1,800 feet, with pieces of wood in the roadway and along the embankments. The biggest piece of all, with nails protruding from it, was still sitting on the steering wheel. As he scoured the accident scene, Elias inquired about witness statements. Somebody must have seen where all this debris had come from. From what he'd learned about the victim's condition, Elias figured this was going to be a fatality investigation.

His investigation team worked quickly but thoroughly; they needed to clear the roadway for traffic, but they would have only one shot to collect evidence at the scene. The location of every piece of debris larger than the palm of Elias's hand was logged for position, and photographs of the Jeep were taken. The team filled thirty bags with evidence that would potentially be useful. Elias was intrigued by an intact piece of matching black particle board found up on the embankment at the start of the debris trail. Road debris tends to get pushed to the right as though snow-plowed. For a piece of wood to have catapulted so high was a clue that could pinpoint where the direct impact had occurred.

Where had the board come from? What had it been before breaking up on the road? Did a driver know he had lost the object? There were multiple marks on the Jeep, and Elias set out to determine something called the "leading point," simply the first point of contact between object and automobile. Elias concluded that the leading point was at the front left bumper, in the form of a pressure dent. The impact of the road debris had also released the hood latch.

About noon Elias pulled his investigators from the roadway. Back at the office they would process all of the evidence: road photos, vehicle photos, witness statements, evidence diagrams, notes on road conditions and surrounding terrain. As soon as it was all logged they would send the evidence bags to the crime lab in Olympia to see if they could match any fingerprints. Unfortunately the process would take weeks because they would have to check every surface.

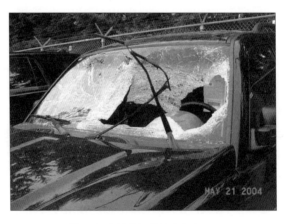

The windshield of Maria's Jeep
Photo admitted as evidence Cause No. 06-02-11563

Collisions usually occur because a driver is doing something stupid, speeding or driving under the influence. The injured driver in this case was clearly a victim of circumstance. The object had come out of nowhere; Elias needed to figure out how the object had gotten into the roadway. He was going to need help from the public, because the young woman was not going to be able to tell them what had happened to her.

Elias needed to initiate a media blitz.

News of the young woman's injuries had been reported in the local media. Elias directed the media officer to contact every news agency. "State Patrol asks help in finding other driver," read the tagline for days. "Anyone with information on the accident on southbound I-405 is asked to call."

And call they did.

Seattle's Harborview Medical Center admits patients regardless of whether they have insurance or an address. It's owned by the county, governed by a Board of Trustees, and managed by the University of Washington, which is why Harborview is a teaching hospital. Medical students accompany the attending doctors on early morning rounds.

On February 23, a doctor looked at Maria's chart in the Intensive Care Surgical Trauma Unit on the second floor, and saw that she was being held for LifeCenter Northwest's organ team.

"Why is this young woman being given narcotics?" the doctor asked the nurse assigned to Maria.

"She seemed to be in pain," the nurse answered. This did not necessarily mean there was brain activity but the patient would need to be reassessed.

Not every major city or even every state has a trauma center that is certified for the highest level of response, known as Level One. Harborview is the only Level One facility serving Washington, Montana, Alaska, and Oregon, and it took just twelve minutes to transport Maria there from the scene of her accident.

Harborview looms above the city, appearing to stand watch over downtown Seattle. Jefferson Street starts at the waterfront and goes straight uphill to Harborview. The neighborhood that surrounds it, now called First Hill, was originally known as Profanity Hill, perhaps because it was the site of the original courthouse or the jail, or maybe it was due to the steep incline to reach the top. Through its clinics and emergency services, Harborview serves the burned, the battered, the left-for-dead, the mentally ill, the poor, and the rare miracle case.

Trauma is defined as major single or multi-system injury requiring immediate medical or surgical intervention or treatment to prevent death or permanent disability. Level One centers have emergency physicians, general surgeons, surgical specialists, nurses, anesthesiologists and other professionals on-site at all times. Maria Federici would need all of them.

Bob called home after teaching his classes. No answer. He called Kim's cell phone.

"We're on our way back to Harborview," Kim told him. "Maria is still alive."

Bob rode his bicycle from campus to the Bremerton ferry dock. His timing was inadvertently perfect; the loading ramp was lifted just after he boarded the ferry. As he walked his bike to the front of the ferry, he spotted his sister Susan's car and his wife's car. His parents had already arrived from Las Vegas and were on their way to Harborview as well.

On Washington State Ferries bicycles are allowed to disembark before vehicles, but Bobby's lead was brief. His family passed him as he pumped his way straight up the street to where Harborview sits above the city. That was the first time he had ever ridden his bicycle up the ungodly hill, but it would prove to be the first of many, many times in the following weeks.

Bob claims that, unlike his sisters, he's not naturally smart. He just works hard. But he has a B.A. in Economics, a B.S. in Physics, and an M.S. in Radiation Physics. His areas of interest and expertise range from aeronautics to astral physics and climatology and science fiction. To help students understand physics he has posted funny instructional videos on YouTube.

He's creating a meteorological data set for part of the Olympic Peninsula—just for fun. Bob deals in statistical probability on a daily basis. When he heard that his niece had been assigned a one percent chance of survival, he didn't hold out much hope.

Robin and Kim entered through the emergency entrance again. Compared to yesterday, the experience was as different as night and day. There was urgency on the part of the doctors that had been absent when Robin arrived the first time. In a sterile little room, Dr. Grant O'Keefe sat with Robin and Kim and gave them the most complete picture to date of Maria's condition.

She had lost nearly all of her own blood, and her body had been without oxygen for an unspecified amount of time; carbon dioxide had been trapped in her tissues and organs. Her optic nerves had been severed and one eye socket was completely crushed. Her jaw had been severed, with several teeth pushed apart and shattered. Her sinuses had been pulverized. There was severe damage to the frontal lobe of her brain. It was definite that she would be blind, but it was also likely that she would not be able to hear, smell, walk, or talk again. Because there had been damage to her carotid arteries, even if blood flow was returning to her brain the doctors could not be sure how much blood was getting to her brain and how damaged it had been while without.

Even more chillingly, the doctor said to Robin, "One day she may hate us for saving her life."

Earlier that morning, on the way back to Harborview, it had occurred to Robin that it was a blessing that Maria had specified on her driver's license that she wanted to be an organ donor. Doctors had explained to Robin the night before that in order to keep her organs and tissues viable they would continue giving Maria fluids and oxygen. They were also keeping her body temperature low so as to reduce bleeding. What if Maria hadn't been an organ donor and doctors had asked Robin if she wanted them to remove life support? Thank heavens she had not had to make that decision. Robin felt a certain peace in returning to Harborview. If Maria had managed to survive the night on her own, then Robin would do anything necessary to keep her alive.

Because most of the Northwest's most severe trauma cases end up at Harborview, the hospital is the source of the majority of the region's organ donors. Harborview staff are trained to identify non-survivable injuries and contact LifeCenter Northwest. Organ recovery coordinators arrive to explain clinical death to the next of kin and take them through copious paperwork needed for consent. There are two legal definitions of death: cardio-pulmonary and brain. In cardio-pulmonary death, the lungs and heart have lost their ability to function and their loss is not reversible. Brain death is when blood flow to the brain has stopped and brain function has permanently ceased. In both cases patients can technically be kept alive by the use of machines to push air into their lungs or blood in and out of their hearts, but without the machine the functions would cease.

If a potential donor has not been pronounced dead, the patient has to be on ventilated support in order to meet LifeCenter Northwest criteria. Doctors perform a series of tests to check on a patient's ability to breathe on her own, whether she has a gag response, or can respond to pain. The coordinators always have to tell family members that a patient can be clinically dead but still appear alive and warm to the touch.

Maria would have been an excellent candidate for organ donation. She was young and strong. Her injuries were primarily to the face, although some upper abdominal damage was noted later. She'd given first-person consent through her Washington State driver's license. She was on a ventilator but appeared to be brain dead. That had left Robin to complete the social and medical history. But by the next day it became apparent that the life Maria had to give was to herself; she no longer had organs to share.

Dr. O'Keefe's comment about whether Maria would ever forgive them for saving her shattered Robin's sense of elation that Maria was still alive. Yes, Maria had survived the night but what was the prognosis? The doctors couldn't even estimate the brain damage. Robin knew her daughter wouldn't want to be a vegetable. The calm she had felt earlier when she believed that Maria had somehow chosen to live had been replaced with panic. What would the quality of her life be like? Maria worked three different restaurant jobs; she didn't have health insurance. How could they pay for her care? It didn't take long for this worry to seem unimportant, like her worry about getting a parking ticket outside of the emergency room. She couldn't afford to lose her daughter.

Most of Robin's family migrated back to Harborview that day. Her brother-in-law, Steve, was an attorney who had worked with the Washington State Patrol in the past. He was in contact with the agency about Maria's accident investigation, and reported that the Patrol was setting up a special number for anyone with information about the accident to call.

Robin wanted other family members to meet the doctors with her because she could not retain all that they were telling her. She needed others to help her answer their questions. For instance, they asked her what type of resuscitation measures to use on Maria. And when doctors told her what they'd seen on an angiogram, she didn't understand the terms they used. Finally the doctors laid out a clear plan. It was now Monday. If Maria survived until Wednesday they would do a clean-out surgery to remove the debris and bone fragments. If she lived until Friday they would reconstruct her face. But they needed her vitals to be stronger before they could proceed. Their plan was a mantra for Robin, and a promise.

Dr. Copass had been Harborview's Director of Emergency Medical Services for thirty-one years. In publications, the word "legendary" is often used to describe him. He was considered responsible for putting Harborview on the elite map of Level One trauma centers in the western United States. Harborview's emergency room serves over 200 cases per day, 80,000-plus per year. Copass also directed the emergency response organization known as Medic One, in which paramedics are trained to think and operate like emergency room doctors. He personally trained those paramedics. In addition, he created and ran Airlift Northwest, the air transport service for critically ill or injured patients.

Trauma centers are required to track patient outcomes, so when the head of emergency services later swears under oath that he has never had a patient survive an injury similar to that of Maria Federici, he has the data to prove it. "It was beyond catastrophic," he said of her injuries. "It was an event."

The first media request for information on Maria was logged by Harborview's Media Relations Director, Susan Gregg-Hanson, later in the day that Maria arrived in the emergency room at 12:30 a.m. People who had heard about Maria in the news were calling Harborview's main number to ask if there were any more information on her condition. The receptionists were not at liberty to say anything about her, but they accepted messages to be passed along to the family.

Gregg-Hanson's Harborview title was Director, Media Relations and Public Relations. With over fifteen years in her field, she was no stranger to stories that caught the public interest. She was new at Children's Hospital during a deadly eColi outbreak and had started at Harborview the same month that Mardi Gras violence and the Nisqually earthquake rocked the Northwest. She could predict what medical cases would generate media attention. Children always generate interest, as do innocent people like Maria who happened to be in the wrong place at the wrong time.

The accident was clearly a priority for the State Patrol. As the news media started to pick up the story, reporters included Maria's name and the fact that she was in critical condition at Harborview. The calls to Gregg-Hanson were mostly requests for updates on Maria's condition and to find out whether a family member was available to speak to the press. It was time for Gregg-Hanson to meet Maria's mother.

As part of her job, Gregg-Hanson, who has a family herself, interacts with families at what may be the most emotional time in their lives. She's grateful that families are willing to connect with her during these sudden crises. A family may plan in advance for surgery or childbirth; no one anticipates traumatic injury. She is constantly amazed by how families respond during the worst times imaginable. Most have never had to cope with life-threatening injuries yet they do cope and even inspire others.

Maria's outcome was still uncertain when Gregg-Hanson first met her mother, but Robin told her she knew she was going to need all of the support possible. Robin would be willing to speak with anyone in order to help the State Patrol locate the driver. Her brother-in-law, Steve Hansen, was acting as point person.

Gregg-Hanson was immediately impressed with Robin. She was incredibly thoughtful in her responses, able to think before speaking even though she had not even left the hospital for the last twenty-four hours. Instead of abating, the media's interest only increased. Maria Federici was a beautiful young woman. Her story, along with black-and-white photos provided by the family, was touching a public nerve.

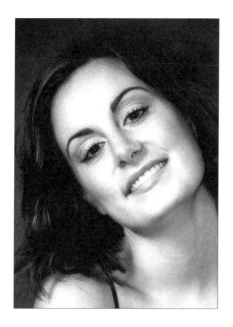

"State Patrol asks help in finding other driver"
Photo admitted as evidence Cause No. 06-02-11563

6

Maria Federici and Kristin Benecke were best friends. While growing up, their houses were just doors apart on Lake Kathleen. In grade school Maria was a year ahead of Kristin but willing to walk with her younger neighbor to the bus stop and hang out together before and after school. For Kristin, this was an absolute bonus because Maria was always popular, and having a slightly older friend in the popular crowd was great. During middle school, they were close. If she was ready first, Kristin would go to Maria's house. It was exciting there in the morning, almost like a comedy hour, as Maria and her mother prepared themselves for school and work, Robin partly dressed and partly in pajamas, with hot curlers in her hair, their dog Artie underfoot. If Maria came first to Kristin's house, the house was always empty, as her parents and younger sister had already left. Much tamer. Kristin and Maria would watch "Daily Grind" or MTV until it was time to leave for school, dancing along, always dancing along.

After middle school Robin and Maria moved to Utah for several years, just visiting their cabin every summer. Then Robin and Maria showed up at a restaurant where Kristin was working the summer after high school.

"We're both going to be at UW next year," Maria said. "We should go together."

Maria had worked for a year after high school graduation to regain Washington residency and Kristin had earned college credits through Running Start. They started in the Communications Department at the University of Washington at the same time, often taking the same classes. Kristin was sure she had to study twice as hard to keep up with Maria, who made school look easy. But it was living at home and commuting together that cemented the friendship. They were still growing up, still in the "I'll live forever bubble."

They alternated driving and agreed on most of the music, like "Boogie Nights" soundtrack and "Jessie's Girl," but Kristin was not a Fleetwood Mac fan like Maria. They found street parking every day in the residential areas around the campus, but if a spot looked too small Kristin would get out and make Maria parallel park the car. Sometimes they went for coffee first and then discussed whether they really needed to go to class that day.

For years they were together every single day, either on campus or on the lake. Kristin loved being with Maria. They both adored clothes; they couldn't ever resist shopping, especially at Nordstrom Rack. Maria always made Kristin laugh with a mix of sarcasm and banter. They loved to point out fashion faux pas among the people they observed, ever aware of unfortunate shoe choices. They were twenty years old, and life was good. They double-dated, went out dancing together. Maria would cook for Kristin, using all sorts of fresh things from her mother's garden. In the summer they laid out on the docks sunning. They planned to be "BFF"–Best Friends Forever.

Kristin knew she wanted a career in the hospitality industry, so she had been working in hotels and restaurants for years. When Maria decided that she wanted to earn money during college by bartending, Kristin was a bit shocked. She was the one with the restaurant experience. She told Maria, "You've never worked a day in your life in a restaurant, what makes you think it will work out?"

Kristin should have known better. Maria had a way of making things look easy, whether in classes or jobs. She was hired as a hostess at Belltown Billiards and worked her way up from serving cocktails to bartending. Belltown, a neighborhood in downtown Seattle, had been a popular place for them to go dancing. Meanwhile Kristin started to see one person regularly, while Maria continued to date. As a bartender, she had her pick of potential suitors. The boyfriends usually stayed friends even after Maria told them the relationship just wasn't working.

Kristin graduated first from the University, and Maria finished up a semester later. Kristin and her boyfriend, Tim, were living downtown and would go to Belltown Billiards when Maria was working. Maria began working at another club, called Medusa, located around the corner from Belltown Billiards. Both clubs were owned by the same person. She was also working at Tini Biggs, a martini bar at the base of Queen Anne hill. After saving up enough money, she moved out of her mother's cabin and into an apartment, above the Piazza in downtown Renton. It was the first time she had ever lived on her own.

Kristin remembers how excited Maria was about having her own place. They'd finished school, they weren't living at home anymore; it was always fun times.

Kristin was at a bar called Pesos, in Seattle's Queen Anne district, sharing happy hour drinks with co-workers when the hostess approached their table. "Is there a Kristin?" she said.

How weird, Kristin thought, there's only one person in the world who knows I'm here, except the people I'm with. That was Tim, her boyfriend. She went to the house phone. "You need to go get your cell phone," Tim said, "and step outside to call me."

His tone was so strange. "What is it?" she asked.

"I need you to do this right away," he said.

She stepped outside and called him. "There's been an accident," he told her. "Maria's in the hospital. Your mom just called me. You need to call her right now."

Kristin pictured Maria with two broken legs up in traction. "You're scaring me," she said.

"I don't mean to scare you," Tim said, "but it doesn't sound good."

Kristin then called her mother, who would only tell her that she was on her way to pick her up. Kristin went back to her table. She already felt numb, and her friends said she was white as a ghost.

When she got into the passenger seat, her mother said immediately, "They don't think Maria's going to live."

Kristin could tell that her mother was trying not to cry, that she was trying to pull herself together and get them both to Harborview. So Kristin didn't cry either. She just let her mother drive without really knowing what had happened to her best friend. Later on, all that she remembered about going to Harborview that first time was that it was already dark.

Arriving there, she knew everyone in the waiting room. Over the years she had met all of Maria's family except her father. When she saw Robin's face, she began to comprehend that Maria might die.

Kristin was allowed to go in to see Maria. It wasn't the machines or tubes that scared her, it was that Maria's face was covered. Kristin wondered just how bad it was that you couldn't even look at her face. She held Maria's hand and then allowed herself to look from Maria's toes, up the blanket to the top of the hospital gown. Her gown was folded back slightly for an intravenous line. When she saw the familiar beauty mark on Maria's chest, she felt like she'd been hit. That was when she finally cried.

Hours later Tim came to take her home. She left Maria's family sitting in their vigil. Then she allowed herself to really fall apart with Tim.

"They don't think she's going to live," she said. "And if she does, they don't even know how much brain damage she has. She might be a vegetable."

What she wanted at that moment was to be able to talk to Maria, because when it feels like your heart is broken your best friend is the one you want to pour your heart out to.

After one day, the lower floors at Harborview were familiar to Robin. She called them the catacombs and knew to follow "the yellow brick road"–a yellow stripe on the floor that led to coffee, food, and the atrium where she was most likely to have cell phone coverage. Most of the facility was a dead zone for coverage, an expression that seemed particularly ominous. Robin had heard that any patient who could be moved out of the emergency room suite to an intensive care unit had at least a one percent chance of survival. But after Maria survived the first day, and then the second, she was one-hundred percent alive to Robin.

Robin had rescued animals since she was a child and Maria always believed she could heal or fix anything. If someone was mistreating a dog, or a teacher at school didn't seem fair, "My mom will take care of it," Maria would tell her friends.

Although Robin had doctored animals and helped her dogs deliver litters of puppies, she was secretly terrified of needles. And now her daughter was a still body on a bed with needles and tubing running from her head, her neck, her chest, her arms, her bladder. She looked like a Martian from outer space.

Someone was with Maria every minute, talking to her even though they didn't know if she could hear. As Robin watched the monitors that tracked body temperature, blood pressure, heart rate, and oxygenation, she kept reminding herself: I'm just along for the ride. I can do this. Neither Robin nor her mother left the hospital for several days. Robin worked for T-Mobile but had no idea when or if she could return to work.

The nurses brought Robin written messages from the front desk. A woman named Jean had called. Her message read: "I stopped with your daughter at the accident. I am praying for her." Robin called her neighbors at the lake and learned that the news about Maria's accident was spreading. Friends began prayer circles that she later learned traveled in huge ripples all across the country, even overseas.

In the waiting room sat another mother of a patient. She wore a sari. She didn't speak English but her body spoke volumes. Robin learned that her son had been shot multiple times. Likewise, they didn't know if he was going to survive. Then a husband and wife appeared. Their daughter was also twenty-four years old and had been in a car accident. The mother told Robin they'd been given no hope; their daughter was alive only because of life support. There was no brain activity, "but she looks unharmed," she said. They let the doctors remove the life support and Robin didn't see them again. But they haunted her. Robin thought, why was my daughter still alive, with so many injuries, and the other young woman was gone?"

Robin was in the room when the doctors made rounds on Tuesday morning, and it incensed her the way they spoke of Maria as though she didn't exist as a person, just a patient with little chance of recovery. "Twenty-four-year-old female presented with severed right carotid, unknown frontal lobe damage," one of them said. How could they talk about her so cruelly? Would Maria really want to wake up if she heard what they were saying? So Robin had the nurses make a sign that she placed above Maria's head. It read: "DO NOT TALK ABOUT PATIENT'S CONDITION!"

When family and friends came to visit, they held Maria's hand and told her about all the phone calls from friends and strangers. The Medic One team that had brought Maria to Harborview came to visit because they wanted to see with their own eyes that she was still alive. The room began to fill with flowers, so many that the staff had to take them to other floors. But each of the people who loved Maria looked at her covered face, her still body, and the octopus-like array of tubes, and wondered, what's still in there?

So many people called the Washington State Patrol with possible information about Maria's accident that Detective Elias had to dedicate one person to log in all of the phone calls. The calls were well-meaning, but didn't provide much valuable information. People near Kennydale Hill were calling to report neighbors who had been moving that day; citizens were confessing to lost barbeques even though they had not driven on I-405. Then a woman named Inge Velde called in response to the media blitz. When Elias received notes about her phone call, he went to interview her in person.

Velde had witnessed what she later realized was the accident she'd read about in the newspaper. Later that night she'd been horrified to realize that what she'd seen earlier must have been far more serious than she first suspected. She had left her home at 11:20 that evening to pick up her daughter at the airport. She was driving south on I-405, just past Kennydale Hill, when she hit some debris in the road and noticed two cars pulled to the side, with a third pulling up ahead of them. The black car in the middle had its hood up. The situation looks handled, she thought. Inge continued on toward the airport, although she wondered whether someone ahead of her had dropped something on the road, which made her more wary than usual.

About a half mile or so farther south, she noticed yet another vehicle on the side of the road, but this one had an open U-Haul trailer attached to the back. There was a man standing near the back of the trailer and his bearing struck her as odd. He was looking back at the road he had just traveled.

Velde ultimately proved to be the only caller with firsthand information about the incident, but she was proof that one person can make all the difference. Elias could tell that she was good with details. He took note of the fact that before she had left for the airport, she had checked on her daughter's flight arrival time. She told him that on the way home from the airport she had noticed at least four police cars and the black car still on the southbound side of the freeway. Velde described the vehicle she had seen farther up the road as a large, black vehicle, perhaps an SUV.

After completing Velde's witness statement, Elias asked her to look at photographs of vehicles. Once she identified certain characteristics, Elias conducted a line-up of vehicles matching the one she described. She identified a sport utility vehicle in a dark color. But what was even clearer than the vehicle type was the shape and identification of the trailer behind the vehicle. It was a long open trailer, and she was one-hundred percent positive that it was a U-Haul.

There were over 600 places to rent U-Haul equipment in Western Washington. But since no one had called the hot line to admit losing a piece of furniture, Elias was forced to check them all to track down the trailer in question. In the meantime the State Patrol had examined enough of the debris to believe that the object in the roadway had been a piece of furniture designed to hold compact diskettes, perhaps a stereo cabinet or entertainment center. If only Elias had another Inge Velde.

CHAPTER

7

During Maria's clean-out surgery, the family stayed in the waiting room on the second floor. While they waited for word on Maria, other worries crept into Robin's head, such as what to do about Maria's car. Her brother-in-law assured her that he would take care of it. What about her apartment, her jobs, her friends who hadn't been contacted yet? Robin didn't realize yet that her friends were communicating among themselves, already figuring out ways to help her.

"If the clean-out goes well," a doctor had told Robin, "we'll talk about next steps." There were so many doctors it was hard to focus on one. Robin certainly hoped they were all communicating with one another, if not with her. Robin had heard they were putting together a team of surgeons for the next step: reconstructing Maria's face.

At last, a doctor came out of Maria's surgery room to speak with Robin. "Your daughter did great," he told her. "Her heart rate was steady. She was strong on the ventilator. It went well."

While Maria was still in recovery, a young woman came to speak with Robin, suggesting that they talk in a private room. She introduced herself as Dr. Anna Kuang and explained that she was doing her residency in plastic surgery with Dr. Richard Hopper, the craniofacial surgeon who would be taking the lead on Maria's reconstructive surgery. She had a soft voice but was very assured.

"We need to have some photos of your daughter," she said. "So that we will know what she looks like."

Robin still could not fathom what her daughter looked like beneath the coverings on her face. Maria was supposed to look like Maria. Then Dr. Kuang did something that no one had done in her presence for days: she reached for Robin's hand and then looked her in the eyes and smiled.

"We can do this," she said.

Dr. Kuang was the first person who seemed at all optimistic. She gave Robin the first glimmer of hope for her daughter's future.

Robin didn't meet Dr. Richard Hopper until he came into the second-floor waiting room on the morning of Maria's surgery. How young he looks, Robin thought. This is the plastic surgeon in charge of the reconstructive surgery, the doctor who is going to give my daughter a new face. He explained how they would need to take bone from one of Maria's hips, and that the head neurosurgeon, Dr. Richard Ellenbogen, would harvest additional bone from her skull. Hopper told Robin the skull actually has multiple layers, like an Oreo cookie, and they would be using that bone to build her new face. Still, they couldn't make promises about whether Maria would be able to breathe through her nose again, or whether they could save one eye, or whether her nerves would regenerate. Their plan sounded like they were creating a Frankenstein, rather than reconstructing a beautiful face. Maria had always cared about her appearance.

"I'm concerned about how my daughter will look," Robin told Hopper. He reached for her hand and held it.

"I have two daughters," he said. "I understand."

At 8:00 a.m. on February 27, 2004, Hopper entered the operating room, where bone harvesting from Maria's hip had already begun. Until now, he had seen only photos of Maria and CT scans. After carefully removing the facial bandages, he took more pictures. Hopper noted that her face was already partially "degloved," a term that refers to removing skin or tissue as one would peel off a glove. The impact of the board had lifted the entire upper portion of her face and split the upper jaw. He explored the injury with his hands so that he could gauge its depth. Since there was no longer an upper jaw to block his fingers, he could feel that the injury went to the middle of her skull, to a spot roughly between her ears. His fingers nearly reached the spot where the spinal cord fits under the base of the skull. Miraculously the injury had stopped just short of severing Maria's spinal cord.

Hopper saw that her facial bones were pulverized, her upper palate was split, and that her eyes had been blown apart, stretched far beyond their normal width. In addition to assessing the injury with his hands, Hopper was able to look at a three-dimensional image of Maria's skull showing plainly that Maria's face had been separated from her skull. Parts of her face had been separated from one another, with the jaw separated yet again. The entire roof of her mouth was also split.

Facial injuries have classifications, known as the three types of Le Fort fractures. It is rare for a surgeon to see a patient with all three types of Le Fort fractures, unless they are performing an autopsy, but Maria had all three. It would require all of Hopper's considerable skills to restore her face.

As the Chief of Craniofacial Plastic Surgery at Children's Hospital, Hopper works mainly on children with birth deformities, tumors, or injuries. At Harborview, most of his patients are adults with injuries ranging from gunshot wounds to automobile accidents, from people who have been kicked by a horse in Montana, or been attacked by a bear in Alaska. A surgeon of the head and neck, his particular expertise is on all aspects of the face and its surrounding nerves, bones, and muscles.

In this initial examination of Maria, Hopper needed to think through the mechanism of the injury so as not to overlook collateral damage. Before he could reconstruct her face he had to figure out exactly what had happened, particularly the angle and point of impact. He also needed to determine the exact perimeter of the injury.

Based on his visual exam, the CT images, and probing with his hands, Hopper concluded that Maria's injuries ended just above the base of her skull and above her eye sockets. Somewhat miraculously, the patient had retained her eyelids. The injuries were worse on the left side, as though she had turned her face to the right to avoid the object, or the object itself had caused the turn. A witness had described Maria as lying on her right side in a fetal position.

No matter what the injury, the sequence of repairs in Hopper's line of work usually follows a basic protocol: top to bottom, back to front. The surgery officially began with the cut from ear to ear, over the top of her skull, so as to be able to complete the degloving, or "flip everything forward," in Hopper's words. Then he used bone harvested from the iliac crest of her hip to fill the sinus area and to reconstruct the skull. Once the skull was shaped, Hopper began rebuilding her face, from top to bottom. He made cheek bones and attempted to place them correctly. This was a little tricky. The cheekbones needed to be where Maria's original cheekbones had been, but they also needed to align with the reconstructed skull. He used titanium to hold the bones together.

This would be the surgeons' one and only chance to rebuild Maria's face from scratch, and it was going to be far from easy. The surgery was like a three-dimensional puzzle; every aspect of construction needed to be in sync with the other elements. For example, they had to create her sinuses and her nose one right after the other. For the bones, nerves, tissue, and muscles to reconnect, each had to be rebuilt sequentially. Even the possibility of future surgery depended on their success in completing this foundation correctly.

Once the cheekbones were in place, Hopper began working on the middle of the face, creating a means for the nose tissue to be separate from eye tissue, leaving a space for eye sockets and to prevent infection through the passageways. Hopper used titanium to form the two eye sockets.

Then he moved down to the upper jaw. The lower jaw was intact, so it was a point of reference. He wired her teeth together and stapled them to the realigned upper and lower jaws, using metal to fix the bones together. Because her injury had caused a loss of blood to her gums for an unknown period, the surgeons didn't know if any of her teeth would survive.

Next it was on to the middle part of the face, placing her nose and attaching the eye sockets so that they wouldn't drift apart. At various major stages, Hopper took photographs, mapping his progress, creating a guide to his puzzle. At least ten hours had passed already. Hopper was tiring but one of the greatest challenges was still to come: the remaining section of her middle face, for which there were no remaining pieces of bone to use for the repair.

The neurosurgeon, Dr. Ellenbogen, had earlier harvested bone from the back of Maria's skull. The bones in the skull have layers, the "Oreos" the doctor described. He had removed one full thickness of the skull, the outer part of the "cookie," for Hopper's use. Hopper then split this bone into two halves, using half to reconstruct the face and the other to fill the gaps. He used more metal plates and screws to hold the bones in place. A young body can readily accept bone grafts, miraculously producing a blood supply, the new bones fusing with surrounding bones.

The surgical team of up to thirty people finished the main reconstructive efforts, but there was finish work left to do. Hopper recalled, "The last two or three hours of the operation was having to bring all of the soft tissues—the muscles, the skin, the cuts inside her mouth, the cuts inside her nose—together in a way that looked like a face and that was working from the inside out. And I was pretty tired at that time and didn't take a lot of photographs."

The surgical team was able to work steadily because Maria's heart and breathing stayed strong and steady. As parts of the team finished their portion of the surgery, they would give a thumbs up sign to the family when they passed them in the hall.

Hopper was pleased. The surgery was going really well. They were willing to operate all day and all night, if that's what it took, to give Maria a new face. In the end, the first reconstructive surgery took just fourteen hours, though there would be seven more surgeries to come.

Robin had been warned that after the surgery Maria would look like a balloon about to burst, skin stretched taut but puffy and bloated. Robin had still not seen Maria's face, as it had been covered with a towel when she visited her in the room. When Maria was moved from recovery back up to her second-floor room by the nurse's station, Robin's emotions were in turmoil. She was tremendously relieved that Maria had survived the surgery, but began to fear what she was finally going to see when she saw her daughter.

Robin had mucked thousands of pounds of manure, gutted fish, and even tried her hand at taxidermy. But she was terrified of the prospect of seeing her daughter's face for the first time since the accident. She was imagining Maria patched together with black zigzagging stitches. If Maria looked like a monster, her daughter would never forgive her.

The family had all been waiting at their base camp in the waiting room on the second floor.

"Do you want to see her now?" a nurse asked Robin.

Robin paused in the doorway of Maria's room and another nurse looked up, smiling, as though to say "You can handle this." Robin peered down at her daughter's face. Her first thought was, where are the stitches? How did they do this? Maria's face had skin. That seemed like a miracle. Robin drew closer. They'd shaved part of Maria's hair and tubes still snaked out to drain from mysterious places, but it was her daughter. The skin looked pulled, as taut as a water balloon about to burst. Robin recognized immediately that the reconstruction was nothing short of a miracle. The smoothness of Maria's skin was amazing. There was clear tape on her face but any stitches were on the inside. She had eyelids and there were those lovely arched eyebrows even if they were stretched by the size of her head. The nurse said, "We'll work on her hair tomorrow. I'm guessing Maria wouldn't want a mullet."

Robin could barely speak. She was in awe of what they had accomplished. At that moment she really started to believe that she was going to get her daughter back–and that it was for a purpose.

CHAPTER

8

By strange coincidence Robin had been heavily involved with administering special needs trusts during her thirty years in banking. These specialized trusts are established for someone who is incapacitated because of physical or mental disability, or chronic or acquired illness. The special needs trusts are very specific in their uses, insuring that funds go directly to benefit the person who is injured or ill, while allowing them to be eligible for government benefits and aid. Robin already knew far too much about the expenses involved in a medical catastrophe like Maria's and recognized that her own daughter would need a special needs trust. She called an attorney friend, John Petrie, to help start the process.

The cost of Maria's hospital bills for just one day would have wiped out every bit of Robin's savings. A week of medical care would have cost enough for her to lose her home. Since Maria was twenty-four years old and no longer a full-time student, she wasn't eligible for Robin's health insurance. Nor did she have coverage herself through any of her restaurant jobs. But as an "emancipated" adult, Maria would be eligible for Department of Social Health Services (DSHS) benefits.

Outside of Maria's room, emergency helicopters landed and took off. Robin couldn't help but think that every landing meant another family being placed in the same hell as her own.

The window was virtually Robin's only contact with the outside world. So far, she had avoided direct contact with the news media, who were contacting Susan Gregg-Hanson every day, wanting updates on Maria's condition. The black-and-white close-ups accompanied every news story and were invaluable for the surgeon.

Robin and her family had been at the hospital every night since the accident, sleeping next to Maria's bed. Her golden retrievers were still at her brother's house. She missed her dogs. Whenever Robin had needed comfort in the past, she had at least been able to be with her animals.

The day after the reconstructive surgery, Robin was in the atrium, the one place in Harborview she actually found soothing. Her friend Bruce was sitting with Maria. He had known Maria all her life.

"Move your toes for me, Maria," he coaxed. "Move your toes." He repeated it over and over, and kept watching her toes to see if she would respond. Her feet were absolutely still. But that didn't deter him. He kept up his commands. If Maria had been able to speak, she probably would have claimed that she just wanted him to "shut up." Instead, she wiggled her toes ever so slightly.

When Robin returned to the room a few moments later, Bruce was grinning broadly. "She moved her toes for me," he said proudly.

Robin was dumbfounded, speechless. Tears began to stream down her face. If it was true, this event was huge. It meant that Maria could not only hear but act on what she'd heard. The doctors had said Maria might not have any hearing. Robin's tears kept coming, but they were of a different kind than those she'd cried before. These were tears of hope rather than sorrow. "She's coming back," she said to Bruce.

The other family member who lived at the hospital with Robin was her mother, JoRene. With Maria's life still hanging in the balance, JoRene could not bear to leave her first-born grandchild. JoRene liked to remember a rainy day when she and Bob took Maria out fishing near the cabin. Bob drove the boat in circles as Maria caught fish after fish. She reeled in yet another and held it aloft as the sun broke through beyond her shoulder and created a rainbow that arced behind Maria. Sometimes Maria was so beautiful it just hurt your eyes. No, JoRene couldn't leave the hospital.

Maria's cousin Kristina also spent a great deal of time at the hospital. When they were little, the two cousins had frequently visited their grandparents together. Robin and her sister Susan both worked, so JoRene and Big Bob got to watch their daughters' girls sometimes. JoRene walked on the beach with them at Gig Harbor and they collected shells together.

One of the cousins' favorite games was to pretend they were travel agents. Kristina's mother worked for American Airlines and taught the girls the names of every airline carrier; their travel agent games were very specific. Once they went with their grandparents to Canada for a week. They set up a lemonade stand on a road that had virtually no traffic. Even after three hours without a sale they weren't discouraged, but their grandfather couldn't stand it. He paid another guest at the hotel to be their only customer.

They called Kristina's dad Richard "The Hat" Geiler; the Panama hat was his trademark look as a professional pool player. When he played a tournament he always wore a suit and tie. But to Maria he was always Uncle Richard. He married Robin's younger sister Susan Abel in 1977, two years before Maria was born. Once Kristina was born they were always together for birthdays and holidays. Richard owned a no-alcohol pool room, and Maria and Kristina would come in to play pool and run the till.

Richard, a Missouri native, had traveled west in the late 1960s for a two-week visit to Washington State. Near Fort Lewis he won a few hundred dollars playing pool and felt like he'd landed in heaven. Then he met Susan and two weeks became thirty-nine years, though he and Susan divorced when Kristina was thirteen. But he managed to remain part of Kristina's and Maria's lives. He traveled on the professional pool circuit but always returned to Washington to be close to his daughter.

On the night of Maria's accident, Kristina called him in the middle of the night and they drove to Harborview together. Uncle Richie was one of the family members who went in to say his goodbyes to Maria on that first night. Her face was covered by a bandage, making her look as though she had already passed. He put his hand on hers; its coldness gave him the creeps. Maria's motionless body reminded him of his brother, whose body he had seen right after he had been hit and killed by a car at the age of twenty-five.

Richard got another phone call the next morning that Maria was still alive. From that point on it seemed he was at Harborview more often than anyplace else. Richard was more optimistic about her recovery than some of the other family members. Perhaps they didn't dare hope too much. Richard thought about how he'd feel if Maria were his own daughter. He would never give up hope.

Every day after work, Maria's best friend Kristin walked to Harborview. Robin called Kristin one day to tell her that Maria had moved a toe. Kristin had been certain all along that Maria could hear, even if they still didn't know whether she would survive the injuries. The doctors had told Robin that she would be blind, unable to walk, unable to speak, and brain damaged. Kristin still couldn't believe it was Maria lying there.

After the reconstructive surgery, the nurses finally removed the drape over Maria's face. The first time that Kristin saw her friend's face was awful. It was more than she had thought she could physically stomach, certainly not what you'd see on a television medical drama. Her face was huge, like a pumpkin put on top of a human body, and so swollen that it looked like it was about to burst. There were no eyes. Her jaws were wired shut.

But after the first time, it wasn't as hard to look at her. Maria was alive, and that was what was most important. Then she started to really wake up, but only to moan and thrash. How could she understand what had happened to her? What could it possibly be like to wake up blind? She'd try to touch her face or pull out the staples. For this reason Maria couldn't be alone, so her family and friends signed up for different shifts to be with her. For Kristin it was draining to have to restrain her friend. Draining and exhausting and very, very sad.

By the second week of sitting with Maria, it seemed to Kristin as if the ordeal had been going on such a long time. Kristin continued to walk the city blocks up to Harborview after work every day. As the details emerged about the accident, and the media fanned the story in hopes of tracking down the driver, many of Kristin's friends would call wanting to discuss the news stories about Maria. But Kristin found it hard to talk about them. I'm in the story, Kristin thought. I don't need another reminder.

No one knows how they will react to a tragedy like the loss of a child. It's telling that marriages rarely survive. Sometimes family members react differently, putting them on different paths. There are parents who need to withdraw in their grief. There are other families who try to make the world safer for others by advocating ways to prevent the nightmare from happening again. Those who knew Robin were certain she would stop at nothing to right this wrong done to her daughter.

Robin had always been tenacious, if not just plain stubborn. She didn't believe in taking no for an answer. As a child Robin hadn't been satisfied with a pony; she only wanted to ride horses that stood heads taller. If she was going to learn to pitch a baseball she wanted to play on the team with boys. If anybody was going to hurt an animal they would have to get through her first. She started working at her dad's bank while still in her teens and bought land when she was seventeen, because a horse lover knows she's going to need land.

By the time Maria had started at Liberty High School in Renton, Robin was Assistant Vice-President of the Trust Real Estate Division at Wells Fargo. At the office Robin always wore make-up, dressed in a suit, her blond hair tamed by curlers. One of her co-workers said she looked like a teenager in dress-up clothes. Outside the bank she was the one delivering manure, shoveling dirt, and riding her horse for hours.

In 1995, Wells Fargo sent Robin to Salt Lake City to be Area Manager of the Trust Real Estate Division and shortly thereafter made her a full Vice-President. While working in Utah for nearly four years, her life was just work, Maria, horse, dogs, and antiques. Each summer she and Maria returned to the cabin on Lake Kathleen for at least two weeks. The renter, by agreement, vacated the cabin while Robin and Maria visited; Robin needed those weeks by the lake.

Almost all of Robin's friends have interests in common, whether it's dogs, antiques, horses, or gardening, with fishing often thrown into the mix. For years Robin boarded her horse, named Mustard, at the stable and home of her friend Louise Cullen. Robin and Maria had lived with Louise for a while before they moved into the cabin. After Louise moved to Alaska, Robin would visit her every summer to fish and fish and fish.

She might have inherited her mother's love of antiquing, but Robin was the only one in the family who really loved fishing the way her father did.

Robin and Maria were opposites in many ways. Robin was blonde; Maria had dark brown hair. Robin was terrified by needles; Maria actually took a course in phlebotomy. Robin would choose riding over cooking, and cared about food only because she knew that she needed to eat. Maria loved food, from cooking shows through planning dinner parties.

Maria liked make-up and clothes that sparkled. She was a social creature whereas Robin would have been happy alone at the lake with her garden and her dogs. Maria's degree was in communications and she'd loved being a bartender; Robin dreaded addressing a crowd.

Besides having stubborn natures and sharing a love of dogs, the two women didn't have many traits in common. In fact, Robin's mother thought their only similarity was a tendency to twirl their hair around a finger.

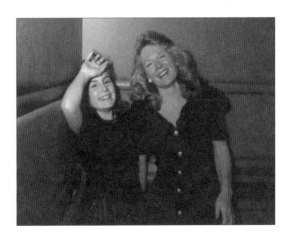

Robin and Maria at a family wedding

CHAPTER

9

When the Communications Director at Harborview told Robin that the media was increasingly persistent in wanting to interview her, Robin could have said no. "You don't have to do this," Susan Gregg-Hanson even told her.

"I do," Robin replied.

Robin felt compelled to overcome her shyness and speak to the media for several reasons. She believed that Maria had survived for a reason. Robin wasn't sure exactly what that reason was yet, but it probably had something to do with trying to prevent this type of accident from occurring in the future. Plus, the State Patrol still hadn't found the driver of the vehicle that had lost its load, and Robin was holding out hope the driver's insurance would help with Maria's medical costs. It wasn't clear yet how severe Maria's brain injuries were, but it was absolutely certain that she at least was blinded for life. Robin knew that providing for her daughter's future would mean asking for help in ways that she hadn't even been able to conceive yet, and she took it upon herself to keep the public connected to what had happened to Maria.

"The media can be somewhat aggressive," Susan told her.

"I want to do it," Robin repeated.

That night she wrote out what she wanted to say. Some family members who read her statement thought she was too forgiving of whoever had caused the accident, but Robin was adamant. "I can't do this out of anger," she said.

The next day, Susan led Robin and her family into a large conference room. Robin sat at a long table in the front with one of Maria's surgeons, Lisa McIntyre. The room was packed with journalists and television cameras. As soon as Robin sat down at the table, people started calling out questions, vying for her attention.

Robin held up her hand and said, "Stop." She felt a little like a cornered animal, but told herself to keep breathing, just as Kim had instructed her that first night after Maria's accident.

"I've prepared a statement," she told them, "and then I will take questions."

Almost as though she had shamed them into good behavior, the media were now completely quiet and respectful. When Robin had read her statement, people began to ask questions, one by one. Robin tried not to cry but she could see reporters who were crying, and it was hard to hold back the tears. They're just people, she realized. They would want to keep their children safe.

"I want the driver to come forward," she said. Perhaps coming forward and accepting responsibility would be cleansing for that person, she told them. It could also lead to insurance resources. "My daughter will live with these injuries the rest of her life."

Robin thanked everyone who had saved her daughter's life. "There were so many heroes," she said. "The Metro driver who managed to get into the Jeep and hold my daughter's hand. The woman named Jean who stopped and called 9-1-1. The two Medic One medics who arrived so quickly on the scene and established an airway . . . . "

Dr. McIntyre's voice trembled as she told the media about how the bones in the upper part of her face were completely obliterated, smashed into hundreds of pieces. But sounding a little stronger, she told them Maria's condition had been upgraded from critical and that Dr. Hopper's craniofacial team had done an incredible job reconstructing her face. "As the swelling comes down, it's remarkable how much of her original face has been recovered," she said.

It was Friday, March 5, 2004, ten days since Robin had been told her daughter would not survive. Everyone in the room held on to her words, amazed that a mother in such obvious pain could be so compassionate and eloquent. Robin's appearance at the press conference made Maria's story even more compelling to the public. Tens if not hundreds of thousands of people would now follow Maria's progress with great concern and sympathy.

10

Along the western shore of Lake Kathleen, neighbors often know a dog's name but not its owner's name. They may recognize the make and model of a neighbor's car but not know the driver. Even though they may chat with one another as they walk their dogs or go for a daily walk, they haven't necessarily exchanged phone numbers. But they will notice if a neighbor arrives home from work later than usual or gets a new car. Small details matter, dogs matter, and so does looking out after your neighbors whether or not you know much about them.

Joan Helbacka has lived a few houses from Robin for twenty years now. The way Joan can judge how long ago they had met was by remembering which dog she had; they met two dogs ago, when Joan's Norwegian elkhound Thor was still alive. Joan would notice Robin walking her golden retrievers. One day Robin admired her garden and told Joan she should come see hers. Then Joan reciprocated and a friendship began.

Beginning in 2000, Joan was flying back and forth to look after her mother in Wisconsin. Her mother died in February of 2003. Friends sent condolence notes, saying "If there's anything that I can do. . ." Joan realized that the more specific the offers, the better, such as helping her clean out her mother's apartment, or bringing her lunch. After losing her mother, Joan felt strangely lost.

Until Joan's husband recognized Robin on the five o'clock news, she had no knowledge that anything had happened to

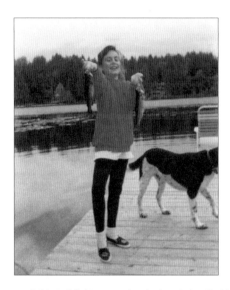

Maria and "Artie" fishing on the dock at Lake Kathleen

her friend's daughter. But she had noted Robin's absence on her dog-walking route. "Joan," her husband called. "It's Robin on the television."

Robin, flanked by a doctor at Harborview, was pleading for the public's help in locating the driver who had lost an object that hit Maria's Jeep. Joan was stunned. How could she not have known?

Joan wrote a note and delivered it to the empty cabin. "I will walk your dogs," she wrote. "I will weed your garden. I will cook you a meal. I will do your laundry."

Robin arrived at the doorstep the next morning with her dogs and walked into her arms. Joan had always admired the close relationship between Robin and Maria. She and her husband had one son, about five years older than Maria, who tended to keep to himself more than Maria did. Even after she moved to her own apartment, Maria visited her mother often, frequently picking her up to go out to lunch. Joan was at

Robin's house one morning when Maria arrived. Her upper lip was red; she had just had it waxed. Joan and Robin were teasing her about the look, although Joan recalls that nothing could detract from the fact that Maria was "drop dead gorgeous."

Nonetheless, Joan didn't know Maria that well. She and Robin had only recently become close, while Maria was in college and always working two to three jobs. It was the same with her son when he was an adolescent and young adult. He didn't want to linger with his parents' friends. But whenever Joan saw her, Maria was always polite, always cordial.

The last time Joan had seen Maria was a day when Joan was out walking her dog. Joan had stopped to talk with a neighbor, whose dog, Ella, was a black lab with short little legs. Maria had stopped by to pick up her mom for lunch, and as they drove past in Maria's new black Jeep, Maria waved a hand out the open window and called, "I love Ella too."

Joan believes there are people who love to cook and people who hate to cook. People like Robin who hate to cook are not good at feeding themselves in the best of times. When their world has collapsed they do not even think to eat. When Robin walked into her arms the morning after Joan wrote her a note, Joan asked her when she had last eaten. Robin couldn't remember.

Joan thought if she could put food in front of Robin she might eat it without thinking. Joan had nursed her own mother through esophageal cancer, and knew that it would take dense, nutritious food to keep Robin going. On that first morning she fed her breakfast, and in the following weeks took her rich soups and stews.

Maria's accident occurred nearly a year after the death of Joan's mother. There had been details to settle and the family was still in the midst of a tough year. Her sister and brother-in-law had both been in the hospital at various times. Taking care of Robin felt like a means for Joan to work through her own loss.

Joan had learned firsthand that strong people can endure the seemingly unendurable but then can be undone by something trivial. During the weeks when Robin was essentially living at Harborview, she called Joan once in tears because she didn't have any clean underwear. "Give me the laundry," Joan ordered. "I think we know each other well enough for that."

Sometimes the people who act as angels in a crisis simply make you blueberry muffins and do your laundry.

Therese Sangster appeared looking like an actual angel to Robin one day in the hall at Harborview. One of Maria's friends from Club Medusa, Therese had white-blonde hair and wore a white outfit as she approached Robin carrying a shimmering gift bag. Robin felt like she was in a dream. Therese knelt down beside her and said, "We're going to have a fundraiser for Maria."

Even though it was already early March, Therese and several other friends of Maria's had a date set for an auction and fundraiser on April 12. "We'll take care of everything," Therese told her, and they did, from donations to invitations, contacting the media and arranging for the owner of Tini Biggs to serve as auctioneer. Maria had worked at several venues at once in the same Seattle neighborhood: Club Medusa, Belltown Billiards, and Tini Biggs. It was this community of friends who rallied to help one of their own.

Therese was another ray of hope for Robin. What Therese delivered to Robin that day was the realization that Maria had not been forgotten, and that very real angels were working to help her. Meanwhile, Maria continued the grueling work of recovering.

By this time Maria had been moved to the seventh floor, from the intensive care unit to the acute care area. The seventh floor is where the family watched Maria wake up physically, but wondered, who's still in there mentally?

The second stage of Maria's recovery was a mixed blessing; as she became more alert she became almost wild. If Maria was in the throes of her own nightmare, during what's called the "sundowning" stage, her family members were experiencing it as they tried to restrain her physically. Sundowning refers to a state of agitation or disorientation in patients with brain impairment due to injury or disease. Although patients can be agitated at any time of the day, there is a witching hour for some when the sun goes down. For Maria, blinded by the accident, agitation could occur at any time during the day or night. She would thrash and struggle wildly, and seemed to possess superhuman strength.

It can be a constant battle to keep the patient from ripping out their crucial lifelines–the feeding tube, intravenous fluids, and antibiotics. The alternative is to keep patients sedated so they do not wake up. However, in people with brain injuries the brain needs to be as active as possible to stimulate recovery. For Robin, Maria's wild outbursts were doubly terrifying; what if she damaged the delicate new framework of her facial reconstruction, in which so many hours of painstaking labor had been invested?

All they could do was hold Maria and try to comfort and soothe her. Robin's mother, JoRene, who had had several back surgeries, even took turns holding her grandchild. Everyone's back ached from the exertion, and there was little opportunity to sleep. Even the floor started to look inviting. All the family wondered how Maria could be so strong. She had never been very athletic or physically active. Robin could understand the inspiration for horror films featuring monsters of superhuman strength, creatures who could throw off constraints while spewing curses. Robin wondered how the nurses could exhibit so much compassion for this alien with her unrecognizable face. There were small signs of progress every once in a while, enough to give them a little hope. But during this phase everyone–nurses and family members–had their hands full just keeping Maria from pulling out drainage tubes, all the while talking to her, trying to reconnect with the Maria they were sure was inside this strong body.

Even though she was physically exhausted Robin couldn't sit still when someone else was attending Maria; sitting in a waiting room chair seemed the position of defeat and absolute despair. Instead she would brace herself against the wall in the corridor, sometimes able to make phone calls, on her haunches, ready to spring into action. Once, when Robin had just been crying from exhaustion, a hospital cleaning woman knelt beside her and pressed a $50 bill into her hand. Robin thought that the woman's extravagant offer was her way of showing how much she wished she could keep any mother's daughter safe from what had happened.

The young patient with multiple gunshots had also progressed to the seventh floor. One night Robin saw his mother trying to sleep on the floor in the waiting room. They didn't share a common language, but they were both mothers. Robin took it upon herself to find linens and a gurney in the hall, and improvised a bed for her.

Although moving to the seventh floor meant progress, the downside was that nursing care was no longer one-to-one. The Abel family felt more compelled than ever to maintain twenty-four-hour vigilance over Maria. She had graduated to this floor by breathing without the huge ventilator that she'd used since the reconstructive surgery. She still required a breathing tube, but it was far less invasive than the big ventilator. With help from physical therapists, Maria was sitting up and able to get to her feet. Soon Maria graduated to taking steps when someone supported her from both sides. They said she'd never walk again, Robin thought, her heart swelling from this new beacon of hope.

Sometimes it seems as if a patient's family, who is with her twenty-four hours a day, knows her condition better than even the doctors and nurses, even if they can't put their observations into medical terms. The family knows when the pain is worsening, or when the agitation level is higher than it was the night before. It still seemed to Robin that Maria had many different specialists working on her, but no one doctor tracking them. Robin tried to assume that role. She also put her foot down regarding all of the medical students who came to observe Maria. Robin felt like her daughter was on special exhibit. "No more," she told the doctors leading rounds.

Another cause of stress was that doctors never did rounds at the same time of day, although they aimed for very early mornings. Robin could be with Maria all night, leave for a cup of coffee, and return to find that she had missed her one chance of the day to get an update on her daughter's overall condition and next steps.

Although Maria's right eye had been too damaged to save, there had been some hope that her left eye might be retained. However, it began to show signs of infection, so surgery was scheduled to remove it. Maria was taken to the operating room and given anesthetic, but she showed signs of distress and the doctors decided not to continue the surgery. Robin was surprised when Maria was returned quickly to the seventh floor. She was having a reaction to the anesthetic, shaking so violently that it seemed to Robin that her face might break apart, loosening those stapled teeth and the carefully placed titanium.

Maria was also moaning in pain. Robin thought Maria might lose her mind then and there. She rang the nurse for pain medication. In response, a doctor appeared who looked to be in his teens. Robin thought, "It's Doogie Howser." He proceeded to ask Maria about the pain, without even realizing from her chart that she couldn't open her eyes or speak.

"I need her to open her eyes and rate the pain for me," he said to Robin. "Why won't she open her eyes and talk to me?"

Robin felt anger threaten to explode. "She's lost her eyes!" she snapped. "And she has a trach tube. Go read her chart and then come back."

The pain medication arrived within five minutes.

That night Robin went home. For the first time since Maria's accident she forced herself to drive past the accident scene. Compared to what Maria was going through, it seemed trivial for Robin to confront the spot where Maria's life had been shattered.

The doctors didn't know whether Maria could breathe on her own without the tracheal tube. From time to time, they would uncap the tube to check her breathing and see if she could speak. One morning, when Robin wasn't present, they uncapped Maria's breathing tube. Satisfied that Maria was able to breathe on her own, the attending asked, "Can you say 'ah' for us?"

The sound of Maria's voice would allow the doctors to assess her vocal cords and trachea.

"Mom," Maria said.

"Say 'ah,'" the doctor said.

"Mom," she repeated.

When Robin returned to her daughter's side, Maria had fallen asleep, but a nurse excitedly told Robin about what had just happened. Robin beamed, and wished that Maria could see her smiling. She waited patiently for Maria to wake up so that she could hear that magical word for herself. Although she was never one for journals or diaries Robin reached for a piece of paper that night and wrote, "I've been in love many times in my life, but nothing is like the love you have for your child. When Maria uttered her first words today, asking for her mom, I knew there was hope."

CHAPTER

11

As Maria entered her third week at Harborview, Robin's sisters organized a schedule of shifts with Maria, to give Robin and JoRene a chance to sleep. After work, Susan would take a bus downtown from Sea-Tac, spend four hours with Maria, and then take a bus home to Federal Way. Then she would get up at four the next morning and do it all over again. Susan was so attentive to Maria–doing things like gently cleaning her eyes and eyelids–that Robin thought she had missed her calling as a nurse.

Robin's younger sister Lizzie had two young kids at home and a full-time job. Her husband Steven had to assume more of the parenting demands so that Liz could spend time at the hospital. The night shifts with Maria were rotated by Bobby, Richard, Robin's friend Bruce, and even Kristin along with her boyfriend, Tim. In the morning Bobby would get on his bike for the downhill ride to the Bremerton Ferry. "This is back breaking," Bobby said afterwards to Robin about the struggle to restrain Maria. "How do you and Mom do it?"

On his visits, Uncle Richie noticed that the doctors seemed so sure at first that Maria wouldn't be able to hear, or breathe through her nose. It seemed that Richard was looking for the positives while others, especially the doctors, were looking for negatives. He always thought Maria had a really good chance of coming back strong. Richard devised a little experiment to see if Maria could breathe through her nose. Observing Maria while she slept, he noticed that she wasn't snoring. But the air must be getting in and out somehow. He placed a Kleenex near her nose and sure enough it got sucked right to her nostrils. Even when he told the doctors about his observation, they denied that it was possible. He delighted in demonstrating the Kleenex trick for them. Sometimes, he thought, doctors seemed to rely more on monitors than their eyes.

Richard took quite a few of the nights when Maria was in what they called her "Houdini stage," struggling to escape from her restraints. He was strong enough to handle her fits, but it was hard to watch little women like Robin and JoRene trying hold Maria down.

One night his daughter called him not five minutes after she'd left Maria's hospital room. "I'm in the parking lot," she said. "Please come down." He was there in a few minutes. Kristina was distraught. She'd been backing out of a parking stall and had turned the wheel too soon. She'd jammed the left side of her car against a concrete post, causing minor body damage, but was as upset as if she had totaled the car. Everybody was trying to be so brave around Maria, but if some small setback occurred, they tended to fall apart easily.

When she visited, Kristin always talked to her friend Maria as though she might respond at any time. After doctors started uncapping the breathing tube regularly, Maria really did respond in her own little voice, sounding a bit like her nose was plugged. Kristin would tell her about work or ask her if she wanted her to put on some music. "Yes," came that voice with its slight echo. There was a radio in the room and they found music that Maria liked, Justin Timberlake, and, yes, even Fleetwood Mac. Within days Maria was singing along. Her past and present were fuzzy, she didn't know how old she was, but the words to songs were still intact. And she knew Kristin, she definitely knew her.

Kristin was working days and her boyfriend worked nights. He would pick her up at the hospital after a shift with Maria, and take her home before he left for work. She found that once home she was almost numb, not allowing herself to break down over what was happening. To think about how Maria might be changed forever seemed to her like a betrayal. So Kristin focused on the day to day. For instance, about Maria's progress learning to walk. Kristin was accompanying her friend around the halls, helping Maria to the bathroom. Maria had always had the smallest bladder in the world, but the situation was worse now. After she was able to speak again, Maria begged constantly to go to the bathroom. Yet just the fact that she could walk was amazing, though Kristin tried not to think about how much Maria had always loved to dance.

Washington State Patrol Chief Investigator Nathan Elias was having trouble getting access to U-Haul records as part of the ongoing investigation of Maria's accident. In response to his request for all open trailer rentals in Western Washington, U-Haul had agreed only to provide information for the Seattle metropolitan area. So Elias asked the King County Prosecutor's office to prepare a search warrant. Still no response. It was unusual for a search warrant to be ignored, so another one was served, by facsimile, to U-Haul headquarters in Phoenix, Arizona. The request would take time, they said.

In the meantime, Elias got a breakthrough. The needle in the haystack had been found. The crime lab had discovered a fingerprint on the piece of wood that gone through Maria's windshield. Better yet, the fingerprint matched someone who was in the system. Elias had a name: James Hefley.

Now Elias was able to go back to U-Haul and have them narrow the search. Within a day he received information that Hefley had signed a rental contract with a commissioned U-Haul agent in Bellevue, Washington, at 6:30 p.m. on the date of Maria's accident. He had rented an open trailer known as the RO model. On March 19, 2004, Washington State Patrol officers arrested the man at his workplace on the charge of hit-and-run, then took him to the Bellevue office for questioning.

The Washington State Patrol's media office sent out a press release about the arrest. Once again Susan Gregg-Hansen at Harborview logged a surge of media requests asking if the family cared to comment.

"Finding this guy doesn't really do much for me," Robin told a reporter in one of her few downbeat responses. "It doesn't make me feel any better. My daughter is still going to be blind."

Finding the driver had brought a new piece of bad news: his car insurance had lapsed. So much for Robin's hope that some of Maria's medical bills might be covered. Who was this person who had not come forward despite all the media attention? Robin wondered. And how was her daughter going to survive financially?

Only days after Hefley's arrest a man in Tacoma broke his shoulder in an auto accident on Interstate 5, as he attempted to avoid a mattress in his lane.

Therese Sangster does not remember the day she told Robin about the fundraiser plans for Maria, only Robin's stricken face each time she went to Harborview. It seemed horrible for a mother to have to worry about her daughter's medical bills when she was grieving.

The day that her manager, Lisa Rios, called from Medusa to tell Therese about Maria's accident, it didn't register how seriously Maria was injured. She assumed that Lisa was calling because she needed Therese to cover Maria's shift.

"It's very, very bad," she remembers Lisa telling her. "Maria may not live."

Immediately Therese wondered if Maria's friend Marcella had heard the news. Everyone at the club socialized as much as their separate shifts allowed, but Maria and Marcella were especially close, had even been roommates before Maria had her own apartment. Therese bartended with Maria three to four shifts per week, and loved working with her because she was so spunky and vivacious.

After telling Marcella the unbelievable news about Maria, Therese drove her to Harborview to visit their friend. Entering the room, they saw a curtain draped over Maria's face. Therese was most stricken by the sight of her toes and her fingers; they were so swollen. There was still blood around her fingernails that hadn't been cleaned off. Therese then met Maria's mom for the first time. She knew who she was despite the fact that Robin didn't look like Maria; the grief on Robin's face was a dead giveaway.

After word had spread about Maria's accident, her co-workers gathered in Therese's small house in Fremont. They cried and hugged and wondered what to do. Therese had never had a friend seriously injured before. Everyone who knew Maria wanted to do something for her; they felt so helpless. The Club Medusa Manager Lisa Rios arranged a lunch meeting with the General Manager, the owners, Steve and Jennifer Goode, and Therese. "We want to do something to help Maria," she told them.

Just tell us when, the owners said.

The news about Maria and the fundraiser spread quickly throughout the hospitality industry and beyond, from western to eastern Washington and then across state lines. Fundraiser organizers contacted the media and placed ads in many newspapers. People from all over Washington began contacting Medusa asking where they could send a donation or drop off an item for the auction. Therese was stashing items everywhere, at her house, in a room above the club. They had a date–April 12, 2004.

CHAPTER

12

Maria was in the seventh floor acute care unit floor for three weeks. Everyone took turns walking with Maria at all times of the day and night, holding her with one arm and wheeling the IV (intravenous) pole with the other.

"What's your whole name?" Her grandmother JoRene would ask her.

"Maria," she'd reply.

"How old are you?" JoRene continued.

"Sixteen?" Maria would answer.

"No, honey. You're older than that. You're twenty-four and you've already graduated from high school."

Then they would start over again. "What's your whole name?"

After the accident, Maria had awakened as a teenager who thought she was in high school, but she did know who her family was. Other memories seemed to come and go. The way Bobby described it, the process was like pressing a reset button in her brain every two minutes; she couldn't recall anything further back. "Great for small talk," he claimed, but still a very weird experience.

They tried giving her paper and a pen to see if written words could flow better. "Kellen is going on a date tonight," Bobby told Maria, knowing that Maria used to fuss over his two boys. "Write him a message."

"Have a good date!" she wrote.

Music was the best bridge between past and present. They kept a radio and disc player in her room so that she could hear her favorite songs. Ray, one of the nurses who worked nights, had a particular bond with Maria, perhaps because he had lost vision in one eye. He was extremely patient with Maria and was the most successful in getting her to move around her room and even into the corridor. You can still dance, he told her. He had her put her feet on top of his. Together they danced as Robin and her mother watched. What a contrast in her behavior, Robin thought. Often two or three people had to hold her down while she flailed; anything to keep her from ripping out the tubes. Watching Maria dance with Ray caused Robin to feel less exhausted, more hopeful.

Maria simply couldn't comprehend why she was restrained in a hospital. She didn't know what had happened to her. Though she realized she couldn't see, she didn't comprehend that she was blind. The eye surgeon, Dr. Amadi, made a point of speaking with Maria to explain why she wouldn't be able to see again. It was a sign to Robin of the extent of Maria's brain injury that she would need to be told. Did she think the world had always been dark?

"Thank you for coming," she told Amadi politely. She then offered her hand to shake, not seeming to comprehend what he told her.

Maria could register pain but did not understand that her face was delicate and newly constructed. She couldn't communicate well because of the wired jaw and the brain injury. In this new dark world she was continually being poked and prodded. She begged to go home in the moments when she made the most sense. She was a wild thing; only music soothed her.

The swelling was going down on her face and the skin was mending itself together, but bruises and scars were still visible. Beneath her skin the bones were still slowly grafting to one another, the rejoined jaw bone, the pieces of skull used to create cheek bones. Maria limped because bone had been removed from one of her hips to use for her face.

Bobby didn't mind taking the night shifts. The nights were a good niche for him because in the morning it was downhill to the ferry. He had always been in pretty good shape, and riding up the James Street hill to Harborview didn't hurt. As a teenager he'd dreamed of becoming an astronaut and always pushed himself physically. But trying to keep Maria from pulling out her intravenous lines was exhausting. It was murder on the back. He thought about the Metro driver who'd stopped for Maria that night and the doctors who had saved her. They were heroes, but in his mind the real heroes were his mom and Robin. They had endurance. It's one thing to be a hero in the moment and another to be able to do it twenty-four hours a day with no end in sight. After Bobby's brief shifts were done, he got to go home.

It was a leap year in 2004; Robin couldn't have wanted an extra day less. What made the last day of winter special that year wasn't that the State Patrol had made an arrest; it was that Maria had graduated to Harborview's Rehabilitation Unit. For someone who found energy through her dogs and her garden, the winter of 2004 had been like one long night for Robin, without access to outside air or patterns of nature. Everything about her life was unnatural–driving to Harborview, parking in the underground garage, the catacombs, the smells of disinfectant and iodine scrub. She was the earth mother, Demeter, descended into hell with her stolen daughter.

Together, Washington State Patrol Detectives Elias and Agent Penry interviewed James Hefley. Hefley was clearly nervous and didn't know why he had been arrested. He confirmed that he was twenty-eight years old and worked for a communications company. Yes, he drove a black Dodge Ram Quadcab pickup truck and he'd just moved into a Newcastle apartment with a friend. What Hefley didn't admit during the interview was that he'd owned an entertainment center or that he had been driving it to a friend's house in Tacoma on February 22. He claimed that neither he nor his roommate had heard anything on the news about Maria's accident over the previous twenty-eight days. He explained that he worked odd hours, fifty to sixty hours per week. He claimed that he'd been driving with only boxes in the back.

Elias said, "What if I told you I had an eyewitness that has you standing outside of your vehicle after the furniture came out of the vehicle? How would you respond to that?"

"I don't know how to respond to that," Hefley replied.

Elias didn't like to see this guy get himself deeper into trouble by lying. "You understand that we arrested you based on probable cause," Elias continued. "We arrested you based on facts that we've developed over the last month."

"Okay," Hefley said.

"We know you were there," Elias continued. "So that's what I want to hear, is what you were doing on the freeway, how the load came out of your trailer, because we have a witness that has you there."

Hefley maintained that he didn't remember anything flying out of his trailer. He had stopped because he'd noticed an extra length of strap flapping in the air.

"James, do you watch Law & Order or CSI?" Elias asked.

"No."

"Movies?"

"No."

"You've never seen a cop movie anywhere?" Elias pressed. "The police officer is able to take evidence and narrows down a suspect because of a fingerprint and things like that? The piece of furniture that we have has your fingerprints on it. How would you respond to that?"

"If it was something that was in my truck," Hefley said, "it might have my fingerprints on it."

Elias showed him one of the evidence bags. "You understand we've got thirty other bags just like this that have your fingerprints. It was a large piece of furniture, thirty other bags. You know what you loaded. Is it just that you don't want to tell us what you loaded or that you're afraid of telling us?"

"I'm telling you I don't remember loading any piece of furniture like that," Hefley said.

"The accident that happened was pretty bad, James, it really was," Elias said.

Hefley finally admitted that he'd owned an entertainment center and was taking it to a friend's garage in Tacoma that night, because it wouldn't fit in his new apartment. After that, his statement never changed regarding one detail: he always insisted he had secured his load.

After one night in jail Hefley was arraigned for felony hit-and-run charges. He posted a $5,000 bail and was released. Elias also interviewed Hefley's roommate and the friend who had helped him move.

With Hefley apprehended, Elias prepared to close the investigation. His job had been to determine what happened to cause Maria Federici's Jeep Liberty to come to rest against the barrier with a forty-pound board through the windshield and a severely injured driver. The Washington State Patrol recommended that the King County Prosecutor's Office file felony hit-and-run charges, but it would be their call. It wasn't Elias's job to have an opinion about what would happen next.

Based on the fact that none of the witnesses had seen the truck and trailer in the same pack of cars with Maria's, Elias concluded that the driver was slightly ahead of that group when the entertainment center landed on the asphalt. Maria's car happened to be the first one to hit it because she had moved into the right lane in preparation for her exit. The black entertainment center was virtually the same color as the roadway and this section of road was not well lit. Those were the facts. His work was done unless Hefley went to trial.

The investigation file went to the Prosecutor's office with Elias's conclusion: *"The vehicle Mr. Hefley was driving was, based on his arrest statement and the registration, a Dodge Quadcab truck which looks similar to a Sport Utility Vehicle. He had in fact rented a U-Haul trailer and had hooked that to his Dodge truck. He had left the Newcastle-Bellevue area heading southbound on Interstate 405. He admitted he had an entertainment center in the back of his vehicle. My investigation concluded the entertainment center had come out of the back of vehicle. Ms. Federici's vehicle was traveling in lane one and struck the object. The object came apart upon impact and the piece of wood went through the windshield and was deflected up into her face and caused the injuries to her face."*

CHAPTER

13

In order to be admitted the Rehabilitation Unit, nicknamed "Rehab," patients need to be able to swallow and participate in several hours of therapy each day. When the medical team first mentioned that Maria was almost ready for rehab, Robin began doing research. She discovered that the leading rehabilitation clinic in the State of Washington was located four floors down from Maria. As in so many other areas, Harborview's Rehab Unit is a leader in the field, "very robust," as the hospital's communications director said. As with most care at Harborview, the unit used a team approach, including specialized nurses, physical and occupational therapists, counselors, social workers, psychologists–even nutritionists. The entire team met weekly with the patient and family.

Although Maria was still a Houdini in escaping from restraints, two of her most pronounced characteristics had returned: her stubbornness and her sense of humor. She could be sweet, even thanking the eye specialist who attempted to explain that she was blind. Mostly she begged to go to the bathroom. Unsure whether her need to urinate was psychological or physical, her family tried to distract her by walking her round and round the floor. "There's someone in that bathroom right now," they would say to her. "We need to go to the next one. Just a little farther. Just a little longer . . . "

Maria's physician, Dr. Kaufman, appreciated Maria and her spunkiness, which gave Robin hope that her Maria was still inside this injured body. Kaufman was particularly responsive to Robin's concerns, and just plain kind. The team explained that to keep Maria's brain function improving she needed stimulation, and they urged the family to keep pushing Maria to do more.

But Maria's particular injuries were a challenge to any rehab center. Patients needing rehabilitation usually fall into a specific grouping: amputee, stroke, brain injury, spinal cord. But Maria had a brain injury combined with blindness. She didn't fit into an established protocol and she never would.

The principal speech therapist was named Ross. What impressed Robin about him was his unfailingly gentle and soft-spoken nature. In addition to working with Maria directly, he trained Robin and her family to work on verbal exercises with her as much as possible. They did word associations suggested by Ross. "Fill in the word," they would say to her. "Night and___? Peanut butter and ___?"

"Butterflies," Maria would always respond. "Peanut butter and butterflies."

Robin wondered, what does she see in her mind's eye? Maria at least seemed able to visualize something beautiful, like butterflies, monarchs and swallowtails had always been attracted to their garden. The wife of the Metro driver who had saved her daughter's life that night had given Robin a journal with butterflies on the cover. Metamorphosis. Transformation. Rebirth. Robin loved the associations. Maria would emerge from this cocoon of amnesia.

"Which is heavier? A feather or a rock?"

Maria always guessed the feather.

The tracheal cuff was removed for good on March 25th. That did more for Robin than the fact that they'd found the driver who had lost his load on 405 that night. When they came to visit Maria, Therese, Marcella, and Lisa told their friend about the party they were planning in her honor at Club Medusa. Maria always assumed she would be attending.

Even if she forgot her age or her last birthday, she always was positive about one thing: she wanted out of the restraints, off the feeding tube, and out of the hospital. She would even offer people money in exchange for her freedom. At night sometimes she would stand on the bed and utter obscenities that Robin wouldn't have dreamed she even knew. But the staff remained unfazed, as though every step was progress. Maria still needed to be restrained at night, for fear that she might damage her face and still-mending skull. The backbreaking nighttime shifts of friends and family continued.

Maria's photograph, the one used by the plastic surgeon, the media, and the Medusa fundraiser invitation, was seemingly everywhere, in flyers, pink invitation cards, and quarter page ads in every local newspaper, from the Burien News to the Seattle Post-Intelligencer.

A columnist from the Post-Intelligencer, one of Seattle's two daily newspapers at the time, contacted Harborview's Susan Gregg-Hansen to request an interview with Robin and Maria.

"I have a good feeling about him," Susan Gregg-Hansen told Robin about the reporter. "I think you can trust him."

The day of the Medusa fundraiser, Robert L. Jamieson Jr.'s column headline in the Seattle Post-Intelligencer read, "From brink of death, Maria fights back." It was the first time Jamieson wrote about Maria, and it was not to be the last.

"Miracle," he wrote in that first column on April 12, 2004, "That was her great-great-grandmother's last name. It's also the only way to explain why Maria Federici is still alive after a freak freeway accident."

To the right of his column was a box inset labeled "How to help," which included details about the Medusa fundraiser as well as a benefit at a latte stand, a special fund at Wells Fargo Bank, and a link to the website, called Maria's Miracle, that Robin's friend Sherry Palmiter created just days after the accident.

Although he and Maria had talked a few days before the Medusa event, Jamieson told Robin, "This will run the day of the fundraiser. You want people to read it that day. You want it to be fresh in their minds."

Between her shifts at work, preparing for the auction, and visiting Maria at Harborview, Therese felt like she had not been able to get any sleep for at least a week. She had never tried to organize an event like this before, and she and Lisa Rios were swamped. Another friend of Maria's, Hannah Harris, had arranged for a donation from Washington Mutual. Therese's sister Jeana was setting up a software system and logging donations. The logistics were overwhelming.

They had run ads in all the papers, but had no way of knowing in advance how many people would attend. Tickets would be twenty dollars at the door, the restaurateur Tom Douglas was donating appetizers, there would be performances, and everyone at the club was donating their time to work the event. Keith Robbins, who owned Tini Biggs, was going to be the auctioneer.

Keith was a third-generation Seattleite and had opened several entertainment venues in the city, such as Romper Room. Once, while visiting Texas, he'd attended a farm auction and been struck by what seemed like a calling. He'd then gone to auctioneer's school in Florida and later organized an Etch-a-Sketch auction at his club. He'd been hooked doing charity auctions ever since. But he had never done one this personal before.

Therese was dating Peter Alexander, a news reporter and anchor for the local TV station Q13. When somebody told her they needed a high profile emcee, Therese thought of Peter. He'd been covering the accident story. There had been an excruciating moment when he and Therese realized that his unsecured load piece was about her friend. Peter was in the process of interviewing for an NBC job in Los Angeles. He'd reported on his fair share of bad news in the Seattle market, from the Nisqually earthquake to shootings, but he'd never felt as personally about a story as he did about the one on Maria. Therese and all of her friends were so young and beautiful. It didn't seem possible that something like this could happen to someone like them.

The auctioneer's best friend was a co-owner of The Garage, a billiards and bowling club on Capital Hill. His friend had connections with the rock group Pearl Jam, who donated what could be the item of the night—a guitar signed by all the Pearl Jam band members. They had been in Seattle recently to do a recording, which was rare in itself. For weeks Therese worried about whether they would really get the signed guitar. "It will be here," Keith assured Therese and Lisa.

Therese knew that Maria was getting better, but once she started to regain consciousness it became obvious how much it would take for her to recover. She would need every bit of monetary support. Therese and Lisa told her about the fundraiser as they nailed down the specifics.

CHAPTER

14

The day of the auction there was more to do than ever. Since the club was closed, they were finally able to tag all of the auction items. Therese's sister Jeana had experience with Challenge for Charity auctions as part of her MBA work at the University of Washington. On the final, crazy day an attractive man appeared at the entrance of the club holding the Pearl Jam guitar. Therese thanked him profusely.

That night was unlike any other in her life. It was a night when a big city felt small because everyone seemed connected. It was a fairy tale. Half an hour before the doors opened, a line of people had formed outside. The club was packed, not with strangers out for the night but with a crowd linked in purpose. The event brought out the most generous side of everyone as bidders competed for the sake of helping Maria. A couple offered their wedding rings on impulse and a bidder bought them both back for them. The guy who'd brought the guitar, Mike Bitondo, co-owner of the The Garage, was there. He caught Therese in a particularly frazzled moment—she'd never done a fundraiser before–and said, "You look like you could use a hug about now." She accepted the hug but cut it short. Even though Peter had gotten the NBC job, she was not going to flirt with someone else. The guitar ended up fetching thousands of dollars.

That night Therese felt like she'd never been so tired in her life. She swore that she'd never do another event like this again, but what she really meant was that she hoped she'd never need to do a fundraiser like that again. The event raised over $100,000.

Bill King does a lot of driving as an appraiser and realtor. In fact he was driving when he heard on the radio about what had happened to a young woman driving on Interstate 405. He registered the terrible randomness of the circumstances and was glad that his own daughters were safe. It wasn't until he was watching the 11:00 p.m. news a week later that he saw video on the story. At that point he nearly fell out of the chair. There was his longtime friend, Robin Abel, appealing for anyone who had seen anything involving Maria's accident that night to contact the Washington State Patrol. For some reason he hadn't connected Robin with her daughter's last name when he had heard it on the radio.

Bill had met Robin when she took his class on real estate appraisal at a community college back in 1992. Robin was clearly very intelligent and capable, but he could see that real estate appraisal, which she had done in the past, was no longer a passion for her. She was more involved with projects such as helping her sister-in-law campaign for mayor or fixing up the family cabin.

As Bill continued to see Robin on the local news and read quotes in the newspaper, he could see that even in the first shock of her daughter's accident she was fueling herself with a new cause, helping Maria to heal and preventing similar accidents from happening to other drivers. Oh, boy, he thought she's going to be like a dog with a chew. She's never going to let go of this.

Bill called Robin. All he could offer her was his friendship and an attentive ear. He'd always known Robin better than Maria. When they'd met, Maria wasn't that interested in her mother's friends. Bill could see that, even as a teenager, Maria was a beautiful girl who didn't seem to go through an awkward adolescent phase. By the time she was a young woman she had the type of looks that swiveled heads on the street, of both men and women. She got attention everywhere she went. Bill knew she was smart as well, but sensed that her dramatic looks distracted people from realizing her intelligence.

Bill attended Maria's fundraiser at Medusa and was stunned by all the people dropping money. It was amazing, he thought, what Maria's friends had put together in a month. During the event, Robin was asked to speak to the crowd. She was fragile-looking, all skin and bones, but held it together to deliver remarks that raised the crowd's emotions even higher. Maria's accident had certainly gripped the public. The benefit was a success in Bill's opinion, but it was too bad it was for such a tragic cause.

Robin was living in two worlds, but the night of the fundraiser introduced a third one, a sort of dream state turned into reality. Being whisked to Medusa from Harborview was like yanking Cinderella from beside the chimney straight into the ball. If it wasn't for the way nerves gripped her digestive system, making her nauseous, the event wouldn't have seemed real to Robin. The Medusa fundraiser was enough to make one believe in a fairy godmother. If only there were a wand that could magically undo the accident.

The club was so crowded it didn't seem possible that it was within legal capacity. People were merry. Perhaps as long as they were raising money for Maria they could have one night off from grief. Robin wore one of Maria's evening dresses, as Robin didn't own one herself. She could barely move, but didn't need to with so many people taking her hand, hugging her. She was aware of news station film cameras and photographers' flashes going off. Everybody in her family was there except for her father.

Robin thought that if Maria were there she would have been over the moon. She loved attention as much as Robin hated it. She couldn't have asked for money for herself, but for her daughter? That was a different story. Maria was going to need so many surgeries, how was she going to survive financially–if she did survive? So Robin just let her worries spill from her heart, along with thanks to everyone who was crammed into the club.

A friend on the lake had warned her not to expect too much from the event. "If they raise a few thousand dollars it will be a success," he'd told her. Nobody was expecting such generosity. The program went well past midnight, late enough for Peter Alexander, the emcee, to anchor the 11:00 p.m. news at Q-13, and then return to the stage. But after the event was over, Robin's borrowed dress didn't turn to tatters and her car didn't transform into a pumpkin. Too bad it still seemed like the bottom had fallen out of her world.

Just two days after his first column in the Seattle Post-Intelligencer, Robert L. Jamieson Jr. devoted his entire April 14, 2004, piece to the fundraiser for Maria and how it created a night when, "the compassion of the Seattle area and kindness of the human spirit glowed." He wrote, "From the beginning, friends and family vowed to stand by Maria and her mother Robin Abel. But how do you explain the perfect love coming from strangers . . . ?" Jamieson was one of the "strangers" who remained forever inspired by Maria, returning to write about her again and again, exploring what made her so special, to the community and to him.

Maria's slow recovery didn't frighten Uncle Richie. She certainly looked bad but he'd seen improvement since day one. Sure, she was using cuss words that no one suspected she knew, and she did resemble Linda Blair's character in the movie, *The Exorcist*, but he figured it was all good.

When told that people were sending donations to help pay for her medical bills, Maria said to Richard one day, "I have money now. I'll give you half if you'll get me out of here." That made him laugh.

Once she started walking, it was really pain-in-the-butt time, with her needing to go to the bathroom every five minutes. But Richard thought, what are you gonna do except whatever you have to do?

He'd always liked the whole Abel family. They were good folks. After not communicating much with his ex-wife for almost ten years, Richard and she were getting along well at the hospital. That was a gift in the midst of crazy times.

Richard was planning a fundraiser of his own for Maria, but his was going to involve pool. It hurt Richard's feelings a little when, at the Medusa fundraising event, they wouldn't announce his upcoming pool fundraiser, but he could understand that they didn't want people to think beyond donating big over the next few hours. When Richard saw Robin that night, he thought to himself that she had lost a lot of weight. Not that she'd been ever been anything but tiny, but now she was just protruding bones and blonde hair. Just ninety-seven pounds, he learned later. It was strange to see her dressed in something other than her hospital wardrobe of overalls and cargo pants, always looking like she'd pulled on whatever was closest to her bed. Robin in a fancy evening dress looked to him like a beautiful bird with a broken wing.

CHAPTER

15

In rehab, Maria's family was taught how to lead a blind person and how to aid someone with a brain injury. But the two modes of assistance didn't always mesh. A person with a brain injury mostly wants to lie down and sleep. Ross, the speech therapist, explained that that would be like "throwing in the towel." During walks Maria wanted to just lie down. Yet she also wanted to relieve her bladder, sometimes thirty times in one hour. It would have been tempting to let them give her medication to calm her or help her sleep, but the drill sergeant instincts in Robin were kicking in. They needed to keep pushing, playing music for her, writing down everything Maria did during the day, asking her to write notes. Their drill and mantra was: more therapy equals more improvement.

Each week the Harborview team evaluated Maria's progress, then sent recommendations to the Benefits department about how much longer she needed to stay in the rehabilitation unit. Sometimes protocol is dictated by the insurers rather than by the doctors. Robin's brother Bobby had been meeting with Sidney Ho in Benefits. Ho had prepared Maria's Medicaid application, which would have been impossible for Robin to pull together. Maria fairly quickly qualified for Medicaid, and it was an incredible relief to Robin to have her hospital expenses covered. Given what the Harborview staff saw every day, it was amazing to Robin how they stayed so helpful. Within days of

Maria's accident, Karen, the receptionist in the main lobby, greeted Robin by name.

Maria had been on the rehab floor almost a month when she was deemed nearly ready to leave Harborview. Robin's sisters, Susan and Liz, began looking into where to send her next, and soon settled on the rehab facility run by the Good Samaritan Hospital, known as Good Sam, in Puyallup, about thirty miles southeast of Harborview.

Outside of the hospital there had been other changes in Maria's life. Her apartment rent for March had been in her purse the night of the accident, but it was obvious that Maria wouldn't be able to live there anymore. Robin's friend Ginny offered to help pack up Maria's apartment. While going through her belongings, it was painful for Robin to see signs that Maria had been planning for her future: books on careers, brochures on health insurance. Robin loaded everything into boxes except for some clothes that she hoped Maria would soon be wearing instead of a hospital gown. Sanders Transfer Company in Tacoma had contacted Robin's brother-in-law to offer free moving and storage for Maria's things; they even helped finish the packing. Maria's Jeep Liberty would soon be gone as well. The Washington State Patrol had released it as evidence; a local dealership had offered free labor on repairs.

Maria had not once left Harborview since she was clocked into Emergency Services at 12:30 a.m. on February 23. On April 21, she left Harborview by medical transport, her first time in a moving vehicle since Medic One had raced her to the ambulance bay. For the family the departure was surprisingly anticlimactic and unheralded, even though there had been so much media surrounding the fundraiser one week beforehand. Leaving Harborview was almost like a child leaving a home where she'd had a difficult relationship with her parents. Harborview had all but declared Maria dead, and then had put her back together again. Now she needed to leave the

Harborview nest and Robin was terrified. Even if she'd needed to be an advocate at times for her daughter, she had never questioned that Harborview had been a strong advocate for her daughter's well being

On Maria's first day at Good Sam, a Covington woman, Sue Roberts, coincidentally donated all of her day's sales from her espresso stand, Le Petit Poulet, to Maria's medical care. Sue collected slightly over $4,000 for Maria, in the midst of her own challenges as a single parent.

Meanwhile, Uncle Richie was finalizing the details on his fundraiser. He'd gotten four pool players, including Johnny Archer, ranked number one in the world, to play each other in exhibition. Admission was $50 at the door at Kennedy High School in Burien. Before the weekend exhibition, Richard took the players–Johnny Archer, Mike Massie, Buddy Hall and local Dan Louie–to meet Maria. One woman heard about the event on the radio and stopped by just to write a check for $1,000. After the exhibition, each player autographed his cue stick and donated it to the auction. The event reached an entirely different audience than the club event in Seattle, and raised thousands of dollars.

Maria had lived in downtown Renton and was considered Renton's own "miracle." A columnist for the Puget Sound Journal often gave updates on Maria and the efforts of groups and individuals to raise money for her medical care. For instance, a man named Don Stevenson collected donations for Maria for his Mount Rainer charity event, in which he climbed to the top of the state's tallest peak. Columnist Mary Swift's headline about his efforts read, "To Paradise, for Maria," referring to the name of the place on the mountain where Stevenson was to begin his climb. Since his retirement, Don had walked and climbed to raise money for various causes. He was inspired to help Maria several times.

The Good Samaritan Regional Rehabilitation Center is located in the west wing of the Good Samaritan Hospital. One of the criteria for being admitted to inpatient rehabilitation is that the patient be medically stable. Robin was glad that the criteria didn't read mentally stable, because Maria was all over the map. But Harborview had deemed her capable of three hours of therapy a day. The average inpatient stay at Good Sam's Rehab Center is twelve days, which includes people who have had hip or knee transplants. The average patient is a 67-year-old male. Once again Maria didn't fit the profile.

Maria was well-treated at Good Samaritan, but she felt increasingly as if she was being held against her will. She would call Robin on the phone to ask, "Mommy, when are you going to be here?" She begged Robin to take her home. When Robin arrived each day, Maria would cry out to her, "Oh thank God you're here." Doctors at Good Sam had diagnosed an infection, but Maria's constant need to go to the bathroom didn't improve. A staff member was in the room with her at all times, which allowed the Abels to finally sleep in their own beds at night. But Robin knew she needed to get Maria out of Good Samaritan. Maria wasn't a frail orthopedic patient or a spinal cord injury; she was an impatient twenty-four-year-old woman.

Good Sam was considered a leading rehabilitation facility in Western Washington, but it did not have expertise in mobility training for the blind. Maria needed therapy for her blindness and brain damage. Noticing that with less medication Maria seemed more alert and capable of therapy, Robin continued to work with Maria's doctors to reduce her medications, evaluating the need for each one. At one point Maria was on seven medications. They needed to be reduced one at a time, in increments. Then Robin arranged for a woman from Washington State Services for the Blind, blind herself, to train Maria and members of the Good Sam staff on using her new cane. Watching Maria walking down the hall, Robin cried. She still couldn't believe that Maria was blind, but seeing her use the cane was better than watching her grope with her hands to find her way.

Robin was advised by a consultant that the best next step for Maria's recovery was at a nursing home or day facility. A nursing home, which could offer only an hour and a half of therapy a day, was not an option in Robin's mind. She knew that Maria needed to be pushed in order to improve. A nursing home might need to sedate her. No way in hell, Robin thought. It would be like putting her in a refrigerator. Yet it would have been paid for by the state. For that reason, a nursing home would have been "easier." But it would have been a living death for Maria. When Robin visited a day facility, she couldn't imagine Maria improving in that environment, and she ran out crying before the tour was over.

On the other hand Maria was just barely stable now. She still had intravenous tubes for nutrients and medications. Because she mostly refused to eat, the feeding tube was her only consistent source of nourishment. Her eyes needed to be cleaned every few hours. She was due for jaw surgery. What had happened to the team approach that Harborview took? Robin felt terribly alone.

Robin had told her family she couldn't put Maria in a nursing home. She'd been afraid to say it out loud, but what she really wanted to do was bring her daughter home. There wasn't a better alternative.

"What should I do?" Robin asked her neighbor Joan Helbacka.

"I have no idea what you should do," Joan told Robin. "But I will never second guess you."

Robin asked her neighbor, Faye Moss, the same question, as they sat in the sunshine on the deck of Robin's cabin. Faye was like another mother to her. She had known her whole family, cousins included, since they were all children sleeping under tents and riding their ponies. Maria would bake cookies to take to Faye, but Maria would also cut her mother's flowers and offer them to Faye for a modest price.

"You know what to do," Faye told her.

Robin's family and some friends thought she would be crazy to take Maria home to the cabin. "You live one step above camping," her friends always joked, but now the words weren't meant lightly. Robin absolutely agreed with many of their concerns. The cabin was too remote, too small. What if Maria wanders into the lake or falls off the deck? How will she get nursing care; what about therapy? Robin was terrified by all the uncertainties, but she felt strongly that a nursing home was no place for her daughter.

As a test, Robin decided to take Maria to the cabin for a visit. Good Sam had said that it would be all right for Maria to spend the night there. Returning to the cabin didn't miraculously restore Maria's memory, but the dogs made her feel familiar and she really enjoyed petting them. Around the dogs Maria seemed to be more in the present moment. When it was time to take Maria back to Good Sam, she cried and begged her mother not to take her back. Robin was torn–her mother's instincts were to have Maria at home, but her health issues were so immense it was also a relief to return her to professional care.

Robin had continued her project management approach to Maria's care, making decisions based on medical necessity and pushing the surgeons to fix as many needs as possible each time Maria had surgery. It seemed more cost efficient to her, and she knew that as Maria became more alert she would fight their efforts even more. But Robin didn't know how to approach the next non-surgical step. Where should Maria go after her stay at Good Sam? Doctors had implied it would be best to put Maria in a nursing home, but had they ever visited these places? The clock was running at Good Samaritan; DSHS had only approved six weeks.

Every family is forced to make these kinds of agonizing choices when a loved one is seriously ill or near death. In many cultures there would be no question but to look after the family member at home. So why did it seem like no one at Good Sam approved of a mother taking her daughter home? Why would the state be willing to help pay for Maria to stay in a nursing home where she would just stagnate, instead of letting her go home where she could live in a familiar, comfortable setting?

Robin began assessing what she would need to do for Maria to live at the cabin with her. She'd need a new deck, for safety, and would need to organize the kitchen. Neighbors and community members were still bringing them food and donations. Her parents owned the cabin; she had almost finished purchasing it from them. They told her not to worry about payments until she was able to make them again. Aside from the cost of Maria's care, they could live quite cheaply. Sidney Ho at Harborview had told Robin about other options available from DSHS as Maria improved, including Care Options for People Receiving Medicaid, which might partially pay for home care. Robin took stock of what she could sell—a diamond necklace she'd found at an estate sale, a carved trunk, riding gear, quilts. She made lists at night when she couldn't sleep.

Faye would often go and sit with Maria at Harborview and then at Good Samaritan, talking to Maria about her childhood. Maria was always sweet and childlike with her.

"Oh Maria," Faye once said. "I'm going to have a dinner party. What do you think I should serve?"

Maria didn't answer for a bit, but then said, "The most important thing is to have really good bread with herbs and melted butter."

Where did that come from in her brain, Faye wondered?

Faye and Robin talked many times during that long spring of Maria's rehab. Faye doesn't remember one particular day, just many, many days, with butterflies rising above Robin's stunning garden and flying over the lake. She knew that Robin was trying to make a monumental decision, but in the end she'd do exactly what was needed. Robin had always worked hard to be a really good mom. It didn't come as any surprise to Faye when Robin announced that she'd made up her mind. Ninety-six days after Maria's accident, Robin brought her daughter home to the cabin.

PART TWO

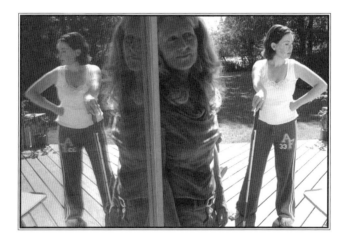

Robin and Maria at home at the lake
Photo by Tom Reese, Licensed use by Seattle Times

CHAPTER
16

The first ninety-six days after the accident had been a roller coaster ride for both Maria and her family; the next years were more like crossing a continent behind a team of oxen, a tedious, exhausting, seemingly infinite ride to an unknown destination. Overnight Robin went from being the mother of the patient to being her primary caregiver, from observing nurses to acting as one. Robin formally contacted T-Mobile that she would not be returning to work. Her employer was very supportive and arranged for a type of crisis package reserved for just such an emergency. Instead of working in banking or real estate acquisition, Robin was day nurse and night nurse, cook and janitor, physical therapist and pharmacist, until she was able to find and hire help. As Robin took on the tasks of nursing, rehabilitation, and mobility training, little did she know that within the next few years she would play an instrumental role in making the highways safer, first by changing state laws and then by challenging an international corporation.

The path to changing Washington's legislation began while Maria was still at Harborview. Robin had hoped that the driver's insurance would cover at least some of Maria's medical expenses, even if just a small percentage. But Hefley, it turned out, had no insurance. Maria's medical bills were astronomical. Charges for the first two weeks reached a quarter of a million dollars; Robin didn't dare look at subsequent bills. There had to be some sort of financial assistance for this type of catastrophic emergency, or else how could anyone afford to survive?

"You should call Norm Maleng," a friend told her. "He's King County Prosecutor but he's also just a normal person."

Robin called the Prosecutor's office and after identifying herself to the receptionist, she was transferred directly to Norm Maleng. He'd heard about the accident and asked, "What can I do for you?"

"I would like you to come meet my daughter and your client, Maria," Robin replied.

His immediate response: "When should I come?"

Robin was familiar with Maleng's name and reputation. With the exception of four years in Utah, Robin had lived in the Northwest all of her life. What mother hadn't read about all the murdered young women whose deaths were attributed to Gary Ridgway, known as the Green River Killer? It was Maleng who decided not to apply the death penalty, in exchange for Ridgway's cooperation in revealing the fates and remains of so many missing young women. His decision provided closure for the families of victims.

Some of Robin's friends also mentioned that she should look into the state's Crime Victims Compensation Fund, administered through the Washington Department of Labor and Industry. It was described as a "payer of last resort," available for victims to cover such things as medical bills, loss of income, and funeral expenses–if there was no coverage from another source. Robin knew that Maria was a victim and there certainly wasn't coverage from another source. This went on Robin's mental list to discuss with Maleng when he came to meet Maria. Robin thought how strange it was that a month earlier she would have been nervous about meeting such a powerful man; now she felt calm about the prospect.

A city is lucky in the course of its history if it has one elected official as beloved as Norm Maleng. He was a hard-working and highly influential man whose work affected more than just Seattle and King County. His leadership on special task forces and legislation made impacts on the entire state; sometimes other jurisdictions followed Washington's lead by adopting similar laws. Although Maleng lost three bids for statewide office, the voters of King County elected him seven times, giving him 97% of the vote in his eighth term. Despite Maleng's Republican party affiliation, he always won in a primarily Democratic county. Maleng, the second son of Norwegian dairy farmers in Whatcom County, wore a business suit and tie as though it were his uniform. He milked cows twice daily during his boyhood days and cherished his participation in Future Farmers of America. He was a graduate of the University of Washington and UW Law School.

The mission of his office was not to win cases but to serve justice. He invited families touched by crime to his office, so that he could share their grief and explain how the justice system works. In nearly three decades as prosecutor he had met far too many people who had been affected by violence, from the families of the victims of a 1983 nightclub massacre, to the wife of a contractor killed on a jobsite. And he met Robin and her daughter Maria within weeks of the accident.

Harborview Medical Center was a place Maleng knew well–personally and professionally. The county-owned facility was part of his official domain, as his office served as its legal advisors. He waged many quiet but successful campaigns to continue its expansion even when construction was over-budget and funds were scarce. In addition, trauma centers act as clearing houses for victims and perpetrators of violence. Both crime victims and the hospital itself were Maleng's clients, as chief of the county's "law firm." The connection with Harborview was also highly personal; in 1989 his twelve-year old daughter Karen was airlifted there after suffering a fatal brain injury while sledding near her home.

Awaiting Maleng's afternoon visit, Robin was anxious about which Maria he would be meeting: the straight "A" student who loved to cook and take cookies to the neighbors, or this demon child who shouted obscenities? Robin needn't have worried. Maria had a few good moments as Norm told her about his student days at the University of Washington. Robin listened, tears welling in her eyes. This compassionate kindness from Maleng made her feel almost weak.

"Why don't we step out and talk?" Norm finally said to Robin when Maria seemed to drift off.

In the cafeteria Norm informed Robin that Maria didn't qualify for Crime Victims Compensation because what had happened to Maria was not a crime in the eyes of the law.

But clearly she's a victim, a voice inside Robin's head screamed. "Then can't the law be changed?" Robin asked. "I need to change the law."

Maleng patted her hand. "You have a lot on your plate right now. If you still feel this way in a few months, call me and I'll help you."

After Robin took Maria home, she had even more on her plate than ever, but that didn't diminish her resolve to change the law to make what had happened to Maria a crime.

CHAPTER

17

Robin had asked Bobby to help her take Maria home from Good Samaritan. It was a horrible experience for all three of them. Bobby was driving, while Robin sat with Maria in back. They weren't on the road for long before Maria started to get uncomfortable.

"I feel swishy," Maria said, panicking. Robin and Bobby translated that as being sick to her stomach.

"Do you think you're going to throw up?"

"Yes," Maria said. They pulled over but she didn't get sick.

Bobby continued driving. Maria, still miserable, cried most of the way home. It was not a good beginning.

Although Maria's first days home were a reunion of friends and family, with visitors almost around the clock, Robin felt terrified by all the unknowns of caring for her daughter. She overcame that fear by focusing on getting Maria to eat. Ever since Maria had left acute care, she had been given hospital food but it seemed to be the same, day after day, bowls of bland dairy products. When Maria was more medicated they had sometimes been able to force her to attempt to eat other foods. As her condition improved, however, she fought their efforts. Robin suspected that Maria wasn't motivated to eat in part because she never felt hungry–the feeding tube delivered nourishment. But the feeding tube was a nightmare. It needed so much maintenance. She'll eat if she gets hungry,

Robin decided. So for three days Robin made sure that Maria had her medications and hydration via the feeding tube in her abdomen, but stopped intravenous nourishment. Instead, she tempted her with real food. Maria kept turning her face away–until the third day. This time when Robin offered Maria a smoothie she accepted it silently. Robin was glad her daughter couldn't see her beaming face.

Maria's first weeks at home were during glorious June weather. This was a gift in itself after Maria's months trapped indoors. Robin's ongoing strategy was to invite her friends and family to visit, as a means of keeping Maria engaged in life. Robin thought that social stimulation might be more effective than some of her medications. Usually everyone sat outside on the deck; the cabin itself was too small to accommodate more than one or two guests. So many people wanted to see with their own eyes that Maria was really alive and at home. Several members of the Washington State Patrol came to visit as well as one of the medics who had treated her at the scene.

Meanwhile Robin was frantically researching and arranging for home care and outpatient rehabilitation. At the same time she was trying anything to distract Maria from the throbbing pain in her temples and her constant desire to sleep, both standard symptoms of brain injuries.

Robin felt like a drill sergeant. "Let's get you dressed, let's brush your teeth . . . " Robin realized that she had always been a rather strict parent, even to her pets. However, Maria had been such a good student and hard worker that she had rarely needed discipline. Now she did. On good days Robin got to be more of a cheerleader. If it would help Maria get stronger she'd wave pom-poms and do cartwheels.

Thank heavens Maria couldn't see the look of surprise on the faces of people who hadn't seen her since before the accident. Her scars were lessening and her hair was growing out where it had been shaved after the craniotomy, but of course she looked much different than she used to. Robin hated to see people staring at Maria. She knew it would be rude to snap at them but it ate at her. Maria didn't seem to mind when people asked her questions directly, such as, "How do you comb your hair if you can't see in the mirror?" Maria would just reach up and fluff her now short hair. When Robin talked to her about the fact that she still might lose her teeth, Maria responded, "I hope not. I'd look awful with dentures."

Wonderful neighbors like Joan continued to deliver food. Two amazing women who'd heard about Maria, Mary and Henrietta, brought over several SUV loads of frozen gourmet meals. Robin was desperately thin at this point; she'd lost over twenty pounds. The food was a godsend. Bobby came over every Saturday. The dogs were in heaven, sniffing at every visitor and begging them to toss balls into the lake on the hottest days. They had missed their mom, and Maria too.

Joan's first visit was the day after Robin brought Maria home. Although she knew that Maria's injuries had been life-threatening, Joan was shocked at her very first sight of Maria. Nothing she'd read or heard could have prepared her for what had happened to that beautiful, beautiful girl. Robin asked Joan to sit with Maria so that she could go take a shower. The sun was warm on the deck, so Joan and Maria sat outside. Maria had always liked to cook and so they talked about food and the dogs.

Every three minutes or so Maria would ask, "Where's my mom?"

"She's just taking a shower." Joan answered. "She'll be right back."

While Maria could talk to Joan about Mexican food and clothing styles, she couldn't orient herself in the present.

"Where's my mom?" she kept asking.

Joan had looked after her own mother while she was ill, but still she wondered how anyone could care for someone with the sort of injuries Maria had sustained. But she knew the answer—if anyone could, it would be Robin.

The days were challenging for Robin, but the nights were rougher. She had set up beds on the floor of the small living room for her and Maria. Robin slept next to Maria so she could wake up whenever Maria did. Maria still woke many times per night to go to the bathroom. Robin, afraid that Maria would bump her face on something as she navigated to the toilet, had removed as many obstacles as possible. Ever since they'd left Harborview, Robin had referred to Maria's "million-dollar face." After all, there were several surgeries left to do. If anything happened to the reconstruction, could they afford to fix it again?

At night Robin's mind raced, trying to figure her way out of the maze of caring for her daughter. Thank God for the funds from the auction, but could she afford even subsidized caregivers in addition to types of care not covered by DSHS? Robin's instincts told her she was going to have to create her own in-home therapy. Not one designed for someone with stroke or paralysis, but one crafted for a stubborn, twenty-four-year-old, blind, child-woman with brain damage, who loved dogs, music, cooking, fashion, and people. But what sat on her chest night and day was the perplexing question of how Maria would survive financially for the rest of her life.

Her neighbor's daughter Kristin was interested in becoming a nurse—yet another Kristin in their lives. Robin enlisted her as a substitute caregiver. The friendship that developed between Maria and Kristin was to last for many years. The perfect person always seemed to appear at just the right time; Robin felt lucky that way. She set up a schedule of caregivers for Maria and, once that was done, decided to move herself into a shed on the property, to work and sleep. It was her sanity.

Robin had begun working with Maria to take her medications by mouth instead of flushing them through the feeding tube. Maria could open only one side of her mouth about a quarter of an inch. Robin was always concerned that Maria might accidentally draw food or liquid into her airway and lungs, a condition called aspiration that can have serious consequences. Robin began to see that jaw surgery to correct these problems should be a priority. The surgery would also allow the feeding tube to be removed, and make future surgeries safer by increasing the ways doctors could deliver oxygen and anesthesia. Yet another benefit would be the freeing of Maria's jaw so that she could start to use her new facial muscles.

Maria had once been comfortable with needles, almost flaunting her vocational phlebotomy class to Robin because it was her mother's one squeamish area. But now Maria had been poked so much that her veins were difficult to access and she violently refused any blood draws. She had to be sedated before they could start any procedures.

As she drove Maria to the hospital for her jaw surgery, Robin thought it must seem doubly cruel for Maria–the always unpleasant car ride was delivering her to a particularly painful procedure. In most types of bone surgery, bones are allowed to set, to graft. With jaw surgery there's no such opportunity. The jaw has to be manipulated so that it will be able to open and shut.

The surgeon's staff had made Maria's follow-up therapy sound straightforward. In reality it was torture for her. Maria was supposed to use a hard plastic mouth-wedge called a Thera-Bite, which can be cranked wider to stretch her jaw and hold it open. But within seconds of inserting the wedge, Maria's mouth would fill with blood. She dreaded the procedure so much that her whole body began shaking beforehand, further tightening her muscles. First Robin and home care workers coaxed Maria to do it religiously, all summer long. When they couldn't force in the Thera-Bite, they began using tongue depressors instead, placing up to eight at a time in her mouth. It was excruciating but Maria preferred to place the tongue depressors herself, at least able to have a sense of control.

Maria's face was still a delicate construction of staples and titanium. Probably during a jaw therapy session, a piece of metal in Maria's face broke loose near her right eye. By a cruel twist Maria could feel pain only on the right side of her face, so she was in agony until doctors could repair the dislodged piece; at first it seemed she might need to suffer for months because they couldn't get an operating room.

When Maria went in for follow-up visits, the nurses seemed disappointed with Maria's progress, as though they suspected Robin and the other caregivers were shirking daily therapy. Robin wished they could be flies on the wall in order to understand how hard Maria was trying.

Robin strove to make Maria's every waking moment part of her rehabilitation. But Robin also thought that Maria would benefit from professional outpatient therapy. So that summer Robin started taking Maria twice a week to Valley General Hospital. The out-patient therapy days were terrible. Nausea from the car ride would last for hours, rendering the therapy almost useless and Maria sick for the rest of the day, sometimes even the following day.

During this time, Robin contacted numerous agencies to learn about their programs to determine whether Maria would qualify for a guide dog. No, she was told, Maria wasn't eligible for a guide dog; her brain injury would make her unable to direct the dog.

Robert Ott is completely blind but that didn't stop him from staring at the television early in March, 2004. He'd gotten home from work and heard the sound of a mother's anguish on the local news the minute he walked in the door. Without even greeting his wife, who was in front of the television, he sat down and listened. He heard a woman sobbing over what had happened to her daughter, and the sound of her voice took him right back to his own mother's torment over whether he himself would live or die after a gunshot injury as a teenager.

Hearing this woman question whether her daughter would survive, whether she would be able to walk or talk again, touched Robert to his core. He had lived those questions, but he had survived those questions. He knew he needed to reach out to this woman and somehow he wasn't surprised some months later when Mike O'Neill, his former counselor at the Washington State Services for the Blind, called him. Could Robert talk to Maria Federici and her mother Robin Abel?

So began his relationship with Maria and Robin. Robert knew firsthand what it was like to wake up from an injury without sight. He could relate to all of the stages they were experiencing, the strong young person suddenly devastated by injury, blindness, and brain damage. He'd been through all the emotions: the pain, the depression, the anxiety.

While he may have adjusted to losing his sight, he'd never accepted losing his independence. Ott has built an extraordinary life for himself, managing all of the food services for Fort Lewis, the third largest army base in the United States; consulting with other blind vendors; presenting motivational seminars; authoring a book and editing two other publications. In addition, he also provides support to other people with disabilities.

After meeting with Robin and Maria, he invited them to be his special guests at a party he threw when he was awarded the food services contract at Fort Lewis. He had a surprise for them. He and six members of his consulting group had contributed towards buying Maria a computer with talking software. A whole new world would soon open up for Maria.

CHAPTER

18

What had happened to Maria wasn't just another tragedy on the news. All over the county, state, and country, hundreds of people took it personally. They started prayer circles and donation buckets, volunteered their time, hosted benefits, and offered their services for free. Maria's accident brought out the best qualities of strangers and the unquestioning loyalty of friends.

Early in July Robin got a phone call from the Prosecutor's office inviting her to meet with Norm and his staff. By then Robin had learned more about the department and its two major divisions: criminal and civil. She knew the Prosecutor's office acted as an in-house law firm representing the county's interests, but Robin interpreted that as also representing its citizens. Robin asked her attorney friend John Petrie to go with her. She knew him because his firm had done legal work for Wells Fargo, where she'd worked, and he'd helped set up the special needs trust paperwork for Maria right after the accident.

In a room at the Prosecutors office, flanked by several of his prosecutors, Norm dropped a bombshell. "We wanted you to know before it's announced to the press that we're not going to be able to charge the driver with a crime," Norm told Robin.

Robin was stunned. She'd been warned it could take what would seem an incredibly long time to decide on charges, but she had never doubted that the driver would be charged. Her daughter was blind because of the entertainment center that had fallen off his trailer. How could this not be a criminal act?

One of the prosecutors explained that after reviewing every existing statute they simply didn't have enough evidence to charge the driver with a crime.

"We can't prove that the driver knew that he lost the unit *and* that it went through Maria's windshield," Deputy Prosecutor Amy Freedheim told Robin. "That would be felony hit-and-run or at least reckless endangerment, but there's not enough evidence."

"What can you charge him with?" Robin asked.

The prosecutors all exchanged a look. "He can be cited for improperly securing a load," Norm's deputy replied, "and ticketed for littering."

Littering–at that moment the word was an insult to Robin.

"What about the fact that he didn't have insurance and that his license was suspended?" Robin asked.

"Those are considered traffic violations, but he will definitely be fined for them," Norm said.

Robin said, "But what you're saying is that what happened to Maria wasn't a crime according to the law."

"Not under current law," Norm said.

"Then we need to change the law," Robin said, shaking inside with anger. She felt like a victim who'd just been kicked when she was already on the ground.

"We agree," Norm said. "But we wanted to explain in person why we can't charge the driver. I know this is very hard for you, but we're on your side."

Robin left in shock. First the driver hadn't come forward; then he didn't have insurance. Now he couldn't even be charged with a crime?

After the meeting, John Petrie told her, "I'm not a personal injury attorney, but you should talk to one." He also mentioned that he'd recently rented from U-Haul to help his daughter move, and was surprised the company had rented to Hefley without asking for proof of insurance. "I'll give you a copy of the contract to look at," he told her.

If not for Norm's kindness that day and John's support, Robin might have been in complete despair.

Advance knowledge didn't soften the blow when Dan Donohoe, media spokesman for the Prosecutor's office, issued a press release stating that Hefley would not be charged with a crime. Donohoe's statement said that his office had considered felony hit-and-run and misdemeanor reckless-endangerment charges against him, but didn't have sufficient evidence to prove either. He explained to the press what Robin had been told earlier: in order to charge Hefley they would have to prove that he knew he'd lost the furniture and that the board had caused an accident. Although it certainly appeared the driver had been negligent because he'd lost a load without reporting it, they couldn't prove gross negligence.

At this point, Hefley still denied any knowledge of losing the furniture or causing the accident. Within the Prosecutor's office a few eyebrows were raised when Hefley engaged David Allen as his defense attorney. Allen was high profile and expensive. Hefley was finally cited for driving without a valid license, driving without insurance, failing to secure his load, and failing to retrieve litter that fell off his rented trailer. He was ordered to appear in court on December 8, 2004. "This is all we could file," Dan Donohoe confirmed to the press.

Robin completed the Crime Victims Compensation Fund application for Maria anyway, in hopes that what had happened to Maria would meet their criteria, even though the driver wouldn't be charged with a crime. One of Norm's staff told her she would write a letter to Labor and Industry, which administered the Crime Victims Fund, regarding the exceptional nature of Maria's case. It didn't help; the application was quickly rejected. Why did I bother? Robin wondered.

By late summer Maria was becoming more aware of her physical limitations, and sometimes she reacted with rage. She would misunderstand the meaning of people's words, and her responses often didn't make sense. She hated these difficulties in communication, and couldn't fathom why they happened. It was almost always words that set her off. The word "blind" particularly incensed her. "Don't say that word," she screamed, as though she were being called stupid. Still, Maria continued working with trainers from Washington State Services for the Blind. The director of this organization had visited Maria and Robin at the cabin, and sent trainers to show Maria how to organize the kitchen so she could cook, and how to expand the use of her cane.

CHAPTER

19

During the first months after Maria's accident, Robin had allowed herself to believe that if she could just get Maria home to the cabin, she would be herself again. Robin had pictured them dangling their feet off the dock together as they had for so many years. But Maria had not been magically restored by the lake waters. Robin could never feel that she was doing enough to help Maria, even though she had found wonderful caregivers. One day, watching a program on the "Animal Planet" channel about Cavalier King Charles spaniels, Robin was struck by their description as fiercely loyal lap dogs. She decided Maria needed the comfort of a dog that could fit on her lap, which their golden retrievers couldn't do. Robin knew that the dogs were very expensive but she fixed on that breed as perfect for Maria, as long as she could find a young dog rather than an irrepressible puppy.

Even though it was Maria who hadn't been able to eat solid food for all those months, Robin was the one who looked emaciated. Constant worrying about Maria had diminished her desire for food and ability to sleep. "You need to get away for a few days," Robin's mother told her. "I'll stay with Maria."

Robin knew it was true that she needed a break, so she left Maria for the first time since the accident. A friend arranged for a hotel on the Oregon Coast, in Cannon Beach. At breakfast on the first morning of her vacation, Robin was looking at a local newspaper when she noticed a listing in the classifieds for a litter of Cavalier King Charles spaniels, plus a five-month-old male. Robin got so excited she called the contact number right away to ask about the five-month-old. The owner said she would go right to her fax machine and send Robin a photo of the dog through the hotel office. The pups were located at the southern-most part of the Oregon Coast, several hundred miles south of Cannon Beach. Before the fax even came in, Robin had started her car to warm the engine. The hotel clerk brought the photo out to her, but she had already made up her mind that this was meant to be Maria's dog. She called a friend of Maria's, named Sam, who had wanted to help in some way.

"I think I've found a dog that could be good for Maria," she told him. "Would you be willing to participate?"

"Do it," he said. "Get the dog. The check is in the mail."

Robin then drove all the way down the coast to Brookings, on the California border. Arriving at the breeder's home, she saw that the kennels were immaculate and all of the animals, including horses, were well tended. The woman led Robin toward the adorable puppies. Beyond their kennel Robin could see a larger Cavalier pup in the distance, jumping up at the sight of her. "Take me," he seemed to saying. "Take me." It was Maria's new dog.

"This is going to be the fastest deal you've ever made," Robin told the woman. She and the five-month-old, red-and-white pup were back on the road within half an hour, the "Cav" edging toward her lap as she drove north.

Robin left the coast for home the very next morning. When she and the new dog finally arrived, Robin could see most of her family and Maria sitting down by the lake. As soon as Robin opened the car door the puppy made a beeline 150 feet to Maria, and then sat on her feet, ignoring everyone else. Feeling the soft puppy weight, Maria looked down. Robin knew her instincts had been right. It was the dog meant for

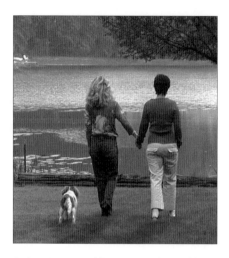

Robin, Maria and Sammy at Lake Kathleen
Photo courtesy of Shannon Grella

Maria. They named him "Sam-I-Am," after the friend who purchased him but he quickly became just Sammy. A few weeks later Robin and Maria were sitting by the lake with their feet in the water, Sammy in Maria's lap. Robin had the mail in her hands. She opened an envelope that contained the puppy's official papers. Robin got goose bumps when she read the date of birth–February 23, 2004. It was the day after the accident, the day Maria got her second chance at life.

Don Stevenson had been dubbed the "Pacin' Parson" because after retiring from preaching, he started walking. By 2004 the sixty-eight-year-old man had logged some 25,000 miles on foot to promote various causes, including support for Maria.

He didn't fuss about collecting money, advising those inspired by his walks to donate directly to the cause. He'd walked from Seattle to Portland, Maine, for Alzheimer's Disease, and from Seattle to New York City for multiple sclerosis.

In August of 2004 he set out to walk the 106-mile North Cascades John Wayne Trail, from North Bend to Vantage, in Washington. This was another walk for Maria, so Don decided to do the walk blindfolded, which he thought would encourage empathy and create more awareness about what it would be like to lose one's sight. While Maria was slowly venturing outside of the cabin with Sammy at her side, Don was averaging twenty-six miles per day through the Cascades, assisted by senior center volunteers and his wife, Loretta.

In August, a 55-year-old woman named Babe Watson was on a business call for her job in air conditioning and furnace sales. She was driving the company car on a road near Snoqualmie Falls when a passing car hit a piece of metal that had broken off a large truck's suspension system. The seven-pound piece of metal went through the windshield of Babe's car and harpooned her face. It's doubtful that she would have survived if not for a doctor who stopped at the scene and performed a tracheotomy, to allow air to reach her lungs, before other medical help arrived. Babe was airlifted to Harborview.

The owner of a local trucking company came forward three days after the accident to say that metal might have broken off from one of his trucks. Babe was in a coma for several weeks while her two daughters maintained a vigil. One of the few bright spots for them was a visit from Robin and Maria. Robin gave them both hugs and offered reassuring words. In the years to follow, Babe would undergo twenty-five surgeries, have 150 screws placed in her skull, retain partial sight in just one eye, and endure constant pain. She would always consider it a miracle that she survived.

A month after Babe's accident, a piece of wood flew through the windshield of a postal worker's vehicle on Route 509 in Seattle, nearly hitting the driver.

CHAPTER

20

Kristin, Maria's childhood friend, experienced a change of attitude about the future after Maria was injured. The carefree days felt over. She and Tim started talking about making more of a commitment to each another. In May, she and Tim announced their engagement and began planning a September wedding. Kristin was adamant that Maria would be well enough to be her maid of honor. That summer she counted down the weeks for Maria. "You have to be able to walk down the aisle," she told her. "I know you can do it."

While Maria was going through the long healing process, Kristin was seeing a combination of the old Maria and a new Maria. She sensed that Maria was definitely getting better. Her face was healing. Surgeons had performed the jaw surgery. Many times a day Robin nagged Maria to do the jaw exercises to expand her range of motion. Maria painfully but dutifully pried her jaws open with tongue depressors. For Kristin it was almost funny to see mother and daughter locked in such a battle of wills. Robin and Maria were matched in their stubbornness. Maria was often cranky about being poked and prodded, being forced to swallow medication and pry open her mouth with tongue depressors. "If you have the energy to be this ornery, you have the energy to do these exercises," Robin would say to Maria.

During a visit with Kristin one day, Maria told her, "I think I can see again." Kristin didn't know how to respond. Maria knew she couldn't see, but she didn't consider herself blind. She expected her eyesight to return someday. Kristin understood that without optic nerves it would be impossible to have vision, but she finally decided that as Maria's mental capacity improved she must be seeing more with her mind's eye.

One day, Kristin took Maria to the mall. She was terrified that Maria might hurt herself by bumping into something. She kept thinking, Robin will kill me if anything happens to Maria. But it was so much fun just being able to do something remotely normal with her friend again. She switched on the car radio and they sang along like old times. It was amazing that Maria could remember all the words to songs with her short-term memory still so erratic.

Kristin was a professional wedding planner, so planning her own seemed fairly easy. She and Tim wanted it to be a big, fun party with lots of dancing. It was going to be Maria's first major outing since the accident, and her first party.

"Are you sure about this?" Robin asked Kristin about the wisdom of Maria being in her wedding. Kristin knew that Robin was giving her an out in case she thought Maria might be too fragile to be her maid of honor.

"Positive," Kristin replied. Maria's accident was what had made her and Tim realize how much they wanted to be married; she never considered not including her. The September wedding would be a milestone in Maria's recovery, but she was also the catalyst for it happening in the first place. The wedding turned out to be everything that Kristin and Tim had hoped for. The ceremony took place in a small park on Queen Anne, and the reception was downtown. Kristin noticed the difference in the way people looked at Maria. If they hadn't seen her since the accident, they looked emotional, almost pained. But those who had seen her right after the accident were thrilled to have Maria back on the dance floor. One of Kristin's favorite photos from the reception is of Maria and Robin dancing. The twenty-four-year-old who wasn't supposed to walk or talk again, much less survive, certainly wasn't expected to be able to dance at her best friend's wedding just six months later. But that was Maria for you.

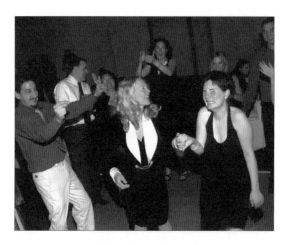

Dancing at Kristin's wedding
Photo courtesy of Benecke family
Eric Sartoris/Northern Lights Photography

CHAPTER

21

When she needed advice on a subject, Robin always figured out who might have the answer or who could help her plan the next step. She was very good at finding the right people to aid her. It was one reason why she had been so successful in the trust division. Robin always looked beyond the hierarchy of the organizational chart. Who can best help? Who will know the answer? Who has the power to change a rule?

"If this had happened to your daughter, what attorneys would you call?" Robin asked a former co-worker in the trust division. Her friend gave her the names of a few personal injury lawyers. Not everyone returned Robin's call.

Robin's path finally took her to the office of Simon Forgette, Esquire, in Kirkland. Robin liked Forgette right away. He was a former JAG lawyer and an expert in trying cases that involved brain injury. She felt safe with him and everyone in his comfortable office suite. He took notes and asked thoughtful questions.

All Robin could tell him was that a man had rented an open U-Haul trailer and that his lost load had catastrophically injured her daughter. Even though Maria was nearly killed and the Washington State Patrol had recommended that King County press charges, the driver's actions weren't considered a crime.

Forgette told her that if he took on the case there would be months or years of work ahead, with only the possibility of financial compensation. In the face of Robin's passion Forgette listened intently to what had happened to Maria. Then he promised to contact her once he'd had a chance to evaluate the potential lawsuit.

When Forgette contacted Robin a few weeks later to say that he would represent Maria, Robin had no idea what had gone into the decision-making process. She'd made up her mind when they first met that Forgette would be their attorney. She just had to wait for him to come around.

After Kristin's wedding, Maria's rapid improvement declined and she became listless. There were fewer visitors in the fall, though Bobby still drove over from Port Orchard every weekend to help around the property. He could always make Maria laugh, but it was obvious she was depressed. For a while after the accident everyone around her had dropped everything to be with her. By necessity her friends had gone on with their lives, whereas she was back living with her mother, reliant on others for rides, for food, for everything.

Maria increasingly dreaded her outpatient therapy. Even though the focus was supposed to be on improving her mobility and brain function, she said all they did was teach her to identify coins by feel and how to make a smoothie. Plus the car rides still made her sick.

"Mother, why are we doing this?" Maria asked. "It's so stupid."

"At this moment I really don't know," Robin replied.

Robin began to feel that that the therapy she was providing at home was equal to the other therapy Maria was receiving. Robin would just need to provide more. So Robin agreed to stop outpatient therapy if Maria would allow Robin to hire specialists for the blind to teach her cooking and computer skills at home. Maria had always loved weight-lifting although it seemed like a contrast to the fashion hound who, along with Robin's sisters, considered Nordstrom to be the "Mother Ship." Robin called the local gym to find out about personal trainers and a woman named Tracy Morales offered to come out and work with Maria. She was shy but did well when, on practically her first day on the job, a film crew from Channel Five arrived to film Maria and Robin. Tracy worked patiently with Maria to build her strength through walking and weights. It was good to watch someone else coax Maria to venture farther and farther from the cabin. At first Maria felt faint and was afraid she would fall, but Tracy persisted in getting her to cover more ground every day. Maria trusted Tracy and they developed a real friendship.

On Maria's twenty-fifth birthday, the first since the accident, her friends arranged for a party in the VIP room at Club Medusa. One of the special gifts she received at the party had its conception several months earlier, when some of Robin's neighbors came over to help her clear tree debris after a major windstorm. Robin's friend Hilary put a CD in the boom box and Robin was struck by the beautiful vocals. "Who's singing? she asked. "That's me," Hilary replied. At Maria's party Hilary performed the vocals for a song written by her father, James Butler, and recorded as a gift to Robin. Its title was "Walk With Me." Thanks to Shannon, her neighbor Faye Moss's daughter, the CDs were packaged along with a beautiful photo of Maria and Robin walking toward the lake. Everyone at the party was invited to attend another fundraiser for Maria, scheduled for November. It would feature a music group called the "Kings of Swing," a beloved Puget Sound institution. Robin's mother had gone to high school with original members of the band; they would raise thousands of dollars for Maria.

Maria's birthday also inspired columnist Robert Jamieson Jr. to write a third story about her. Recalling the fact that she wasn't supposed to survive, Jamieson wrote, "But some people do not know the size of the fight in tiny Maria Federici."

Robin met with Leesa Manion in the Prosecutor's office to let her know that she was ready to go to work on changing the law that kept what happened to Maria from being classified as a crime. Manion told her, "Norm doesn't usually work directly with families on legislation."

"Please just tell Norm that I was here," Robin told her.

Robin wasn't surprised when she heard back from his office within a few days. Her friend Sherry Palmiter had already helped Robin create a mission statement and action items for a foundation to promote road safety.

Norm Maleng was nothing if not a man of his word. After their October meeting, his office set to work drafting a policy paper for the legislature and lining up letters of support from other agencies. The paper was entitled "Improperly Secured Vehicle Loads Are Dangerous and Can Be Deadly." The proposed bill would amend the Revised Code of Washington (RCW) 46.61.655, specifically a section called "Dropping Load, other materials," so that it would be a gross misdemeanor when part of an unsecured load flies off a vehicle and seriously injures a person. The Prosecutor's office proposed dividing the statute into three parts based on the severity of the crime: first degree (gross misdemeanor) if it caused bodily injury; second degree (misdemeanor) if it caused property damage; and third degree (an infraction) for anyone who simply didn't secure their load.

"We'll get this to the legislature," Norm told Robin after the paper was finished. "But you'll need to testify and then get out the message when it's approved."

"I promise," Robin told him.

"I'll be at your side every step of the way," he told her. Robin felt as if he were her rock, her mentor and guardian angel.

On December 8, Hefley was sentenced in a Bellevue traffic court. Robin was there along with two State Patrol officers and Mary Kirschner, the Crime Victims Compensation liaison from the Prosecutor's office. They all sat together. The press knew she was in the courtroom, but what mattered more to Robin was that Hefley and the judge knew that the victim was represented. Before the proceedings began, Robin thought how it would be easier to accept what had happened to Maria if there had been a villain or at least someone willing to take responsibility for the accident. The ordinary-looking man standing before the judge was neither; he was just a tallish, rather soft-looking man. Perhaps if he stood up straighter or could look her in the eye he would have made a better impression. Surely he knew who she was, as if the State Patrol officers in their uniforms on either side of her weren't a clue.

The judge, Janet Garrow, was less than impressed by the driver's request to reduce his fines, even though he admitted to failing to properly secure his load. Garrow pronounced him guilty on all four driving infractions and fined him $834.50. In that Bellevue courtroom in December, Robin knew that no matter how long it took, Maria would have her day in court.

CHAPTER

22

The Abels almost always spent the Christmas holiday together, with Robin's dad acting as photographer, a role he'd assumed after his own father's death. Since Bob's retirement he'd sorted years' worth of snapshots and made a point of sending them to their subjects for birthdays and Christmases. There were always lots of presents underneath the tree for the cousins on Christmas morning. As the years went by, cards from Bob Abel would feature an earlier Christmas. "Look at the beautiful Abel girls," he wrote beneath one photo.

Christmas 2004 was going to be different. Maria was scheduled for another surgery on Christmas Eve that would lay groundwork for eye prosthetics in the future by creating new sockets. But Robin thought other problems needed to be addressed first. Maria had broken her nose twice since the first reconstruction, both times by walking into hard surfaces. Bone had separated from a metal plate in her face and was causing the tissue around her eyes to swell. Also, the muscles supporting Maria's temples had atrophied. So Robin believed that the doctors should fix her broken nose and build up the temples before they did the eyes. Robin also recognized that as Maria regained her strength she would start resisting further procedures. Therefore, anytime Maria had surgery it should address as many needs as possible, especially because they would need to "flip the face" forward again for this work.

During an office visit Robin made these suggestions to Dr. Hopper, who readily agreed. When she mentioned the temples, he suggested implants similar to those used for breasts. Robin was stunned because she'd thought he'd dismiss her ideas. She realized no one would have thought to bundle or change the order of the surgeries if she hadn't spoken out. Good job Robin, she told herself.

Robin and Maria met with Hopper just before the surgery. They had seen him several times since he first reconstructed Maria's face, but during those visits Maria had always stayed nearly mute, head down. Looking at his handsome face, Robin thought back to their first meeting, when he'd told her had two daughters of his own. He asked Maria directly if she had any questions.

Maria puffed her chest a bit and lowered her chin down toward first one breast and then the other, before looking straight at Hopper. "Could you do a lift and separate?"

Robin and Hopper were both startled. Then they broke into laughter. Hopper hadn't seen Maria's sense of humor before.

"That's not my specialty area," he said with a smile.

Norm Maleng contacted Robin before the holidays because he had secured two strong sponsors for the proposed bill, one in the Senate and one in the House, one a Republican and the other a Democrat. Since the process of proposing legislation involved countering opposition beforehand, Norm's right hand man, Chief of Staff Dan Satterberg, had been meeting with various industry groups. It was important to have organizations such as the Washington Trucking Association understand why the bill would not cause them hardship. The proposed bill was on track to be entered into the queue at the beginning of the 59th Legislature, right after Christmas.

Robin thought about how much her life had changed in a year. A surgery on Christmas Eve was a tremendous gift; she was working on legislation to change state law; she had hired personal injury attorneys to try to give her daughter a secure future. It was surreal, yet Robin felt like she'd never been so grateful, at least not since they'd first saved Maria's life.

After Maria's surgery, her doctors announced that the new nose was healing beautifully, with no signs of infection. "Oh Mommy," Maria said one night as Robin rubbed her back. "If it wasn't for you I wouldn't even be alive." It was finally a new year, a better year.

Norm Maleng was a trusted and devoted public official. Given his job responsibilities, people who didn't know him might think that he couldn't separate his working life from his life at home. But they would be wrong. He didn't even have an office at home. On nights without a meeting he was always home for dinner. He preferred to keep his worlds separate, linked only by his commitment to both of them, one at a time. Norm was there for every one of his children's dance recitals or Little League games, and when his daughter Karen died, he was the one who kept Judy going.

Karen had been responsible, like her dad. At the age of twelve she had a babysitting business called "Sitter with the Art Bag." She brought books and art supplies to teach kids drawing.

It was on a "No School" day that the tragedy happened. Not only had it snowed but the temperature had plummeted and many roads were completely iced. The Malengs lived close to a park and good sledding hills. Sometimes Seattle goes an entire winter without a snowstorm; kids always take to the streets when it snows. It was late afternoon when Karen called from a friend's house, saying they were going to McGraw hill.

Judy still plays the phone call over in her mind. "No," she told her daughter, "dad is picking you up at Shelly's house at five o'clock." But Karen was insistent, and Judy finally gave in.

"Fine," she finally said.

A short time later, as Judy started reading a book she'd received for Christmas, she thought how strangely quiet it seemed; icy streets were keeping drivers at home. Suddenly the phone rang and a voice said, "Karen's been in an accident."

Judy drove cautiously to a nearby church where three girls were being treated by firefighters. Karen was unconscious. What had happened? Karen and two friends were sledding down McGraw on an inner tube when a car drove into the intersection. Karen's head hit the car bumper while the other girls were thrown clear. A medical helicopter soon landed at the park a few blocks away. Judy learned later that the airlift helicopter had never been used within the city limits, but the roads were nearly impassable due to ice. The doctor who jumped out of the helicopter to treat the girls was Dr. Michael Copass, head of Harborview's Emergency Services. He had been the first one to grab a bag and get on the helicopter.

Later that night at Harborview Hospital, Norm held Judy as she sobbed outside the emergency room. Doctors had confirmed they couldn't save Karen. The cause of death was brain injury.

In the dark days that followed, it was Norm who managed to function as a parent, making dinner for their younger son Mark, helping with his homework. There were times when Judy felt like she couldn't get out of bed. Norm's sorrow was obvious; he wore it on his face. But he managed to go to work as always, and was as constant as the day. For months Judy found herself listening for Karen at night, thinking the sound of a car door meant she was home late from babysitting.

After six months, Judy enrolled in the MBA program at Seattle University; at graduation she requested that her diploma include Karen's name, to honor her memory. Her friends assumed that she might become overly protective of Mark. Instead she encouraged him to live life to the fullest.

Norm said yes to more requests at work. Governor Booth Gardner asked him to take part in a Community Protection Task Force. Norm became even more committed to protecting other people, especially children. Sometimes people who have suffered a loss don't think that anyone else can understand what they are going through unless they have experienced a loss of their own. Judy believed this, but worried that Norm took every subsequent loss more personally.

Early in Norm's career he was on staff in the Washington, D.C., office of Washington's Senator Warren Magnuson. One of his duties was to work on passing the Flammable Fabrics Act, a legislative response to prevent children from being burned because of nightwear. The act was ultimately signed into law by President Lyndon Johnson. After joining the King County Prosecutor's office in 1971 as Chief of the Civil Division, Norm created a Special Assault Unit—the first in the nation to deal exclusively with the sexual and physical abuse of children. In 1978, voters elected him to be King County Prosecutor. By 1981 his office had brought out drug-law reform that was later hailed in the Washington Law Review as "the most comprehensive sentencing reform measure enacted in the U.S. in 50 years."

From protecting children from sexual abuse to enacting criminal sentencing reform, Norm was particularly drawn to help those who couldn't protect themselves. Shortly after Maria's accident, Norm had told Judy about visiting the young woman at Harborview. Maria was twenty-four years old, three years younger than Karen would have been had she lived. Judy wasn't surprised when Norm began working closely with Maria's mother to change the unsecured load law. Maria was a beautiful young woman who'd had no chance of protecting herself, plus she had suffered a brain injury and been treated at Harborview.

The letter from Norm to Representative Ruth Kagi asking her to sponsor the bill to amend RCW 46.61.155 was a formality. Norm and Ruth had already spoken at length about her sponsorship, agreeing that her colleague, Representative Al O'Brien, should take the committee lead. Norm and Ruth's working relationship went back many years; they had logged days if not months together on the Sentencing Guidelines Commission, attending community meetings across the state. Norm had insisted on going to all of them. When his children Karen and Mark were young they'd ask him, "What did you do at work Daddy?"

"Meetings," he told them. "Just meetings."

CHAPTER

23

Learning the legislative process was another crash course for Robin. But she was a fast learner. Bills need to pass in both the House of Representatives and the Senate. What are called "companion" bills are introduced at the same time in both houses. Norm had found sponsors for each. Luke Esser, 48th District, was going to be the Senate sponsor and Ruth Kagi, 32nd District, would sponsor the bill in the House. Once the bills were introduced they would go "to committee" for further study.

Although raised in Washington state, Robin had never once visited the Capitol building in Olympia before the day she met Luke Esser. Compared to Seattle or Tacoma, Olympia is small, dominated by government offices. Those who take the popular Capital building tour learn such trivia as the dome that sits atop it is the fourth tallest in the world. The State Senate is on one side of the dome, the House of Representatives on the other. Robin quickly learned about the cafeteria in the library, where she found refuge during the many long days she spent at the Capitol. Robin also learned that some 2,400 bills are introduced each year in the House and Senate combined; on average only 500 are enacted. Robin was hell bent that their bill would be one of those 500 in 2005. "Never underestimate the power of a pissed-off mom," she'd say when her friends questioned taking on a cause beyond Maria's recovery, but in truth she never let anyone see her anger, just her determination.

While in committee, proposed bills are studied, sometimes in joint meetings between the House and Senate. Each committee reviews letters from state agencies and holds public hearings in order to hear testimony. Then the committee votes on whether to advance the bill to the full legislature. Robin was astounded when she learned the date for the public hearing on what was officially known as Senate Bill 5457. It was scheduled for February 23, 2005: the one-year anniversary of when Robin was called back to Harborview–the date Maria considered her new birthday.

Representative Ruth Kagi's first term in the Washington State Legislature started on January 1, 2001. Ruth's district, the 32nd, was in the area north of Seattle that included Lake Forest Park. Within a year she was working closely with Norm Maleng on part of the drug sentencing reform bill for the 2002 session. Kagi considered Norm a remarkable man who was always bipartisan. She attended many community meetings with him. He listened to every word spoken, and considered each idea carefully before responding. The sentencing reform they ultimately proposed to the legislature was not going to be popular among Norm's fellow Republicans, but Norm always cared more about doing what was right than what was popular. The journey to passing that legislation was long and arduous. Kagi knew the drug bill would not have succeeded except for Norm's calm perseverance.

When Norm asked Kagi to be the prime sponsor of the bill to increase criminal penalties for driving with an unsecured load, she agreed without hesitation. She had heard about Maria's accident. As the mother of step-sons and two daughters, she could easily imagine another mother's pain. The accident struck her as one that could have been prevented, and that made it even more tragic. Kagi wondered, it could have happened to anyone, but what if it happened to my daughter?

Ruth also knew that Norm had done most of the hard work already, producing a white paper and drafting the bill's language. He promised ongoing support through the 2005 session; he or Chief of Staff Satterberg would communicate with committee chairs and he was already making phone calls to line up backers. She was happy, *happy* to take it on. The proposed bill didn't have a fiscal impact so it should pass easier than those that do. And who could be against requiring drivers to secure their loads to prevent road debris that was expensive to remove and potentially deadly?

Little did Representative Kagi know that her agreement to sponsor the bill in the House was the beginning of a journey that would become highly personal.

Given a choice, Robin would always choose to pull on comfortable clothes from beside her bed to put on the next morning. She liked finding the occasional vintage stole or jewelry at an estate sale, but she really could care less about clothes. Ever since childhood days, when she just wanted to help her father build something, fish, or ride her horse, Robin preferred clothes that let her muck out stalls, get muddy with the dogs, and stay warm. But as an adult, she'd worked for banks and corporations, and had a mother who still turned heads in her eighties. Robin knew how to play the appearance game, wear the pantyhose, tame her hair. She couldn't testify in Olympia looking like she'd just been rolling in the garden with the dogs. She went for her banker's look in a light-colored suit.

Robin, Maria, and Maria's caregiver and friend, Kristin, all went to Olympia for the Judicial Committee hearing. Maria held her head and moaned on the way. Robin tried not to be too distracted by all the unsecured loads she noticed on the forty-mile drive.

"I'm going to throw up," Maria said.

"Breathe," Robin told her. "Breathe."

At the Capitol, Norm greeted Maria and Robin, and sat with them while they waited outside the huge conference room where the Judicial Committee was scheduled to meet. All of Robin's family arrived. Norm patted Robin's hand the way he had the very first time they'd met.

"You'll do great," he told her.

Entering the conference room, Robin and Norm took their places together behind a long table. Norm testified first. It gave Robin courage hearing him make such a strong case for the legislation in front of the committee. He concluded by calling on Washington State "to become a leader in elevating unsecured loads to a gross misdemeanor in cases of bodily harm." Then Norm moved the microphone over to Robin and gave her hand a squeeze.

"My name is Robin Abel," she started. "On February 22, 2004, I received the call that is every parent's worst nightmare. It was Harborview Hospital. This woman said to me. 'Is your daughter Maria Federici?'"

Her voice started to tremble as she told about rushing to the emergency room. She wasn't sure she could continue without crying. So she looked at Norm and he smiled at her. She took a breath and continued, "'Are you here for her organs?' I asked the doctors when they came to speak with me, and they nodded yes."

All the committee members facing Robin were paying rapt attention. She knew that Maria and all of her family were sitting behind her. "My daughter will need care for the rest of her life... this law is to prevent what happened to my daughter from happening to yours."

After the session was adjourned, Bobby told Robin. "I have never been so proud of you. You saved lives today!" Robin's testimony was powerful.

Later that day, the committee voted unanimously to send the bill towards a full senate vote. "That's extraordinary," Senator Esser told Robin. "It's very unusual to pass a bill so quickly." Another senator commented to Robin, "You couldn't have a better guardian angel than Norm."

After Robin's testimony before the Senate Judicial Committee, Representative Kagi met Robin and Maria for the first time. Kagi was immediately impressed by Robin's understanding of the legislative process and her personal drive. Robin already understood that the legislation, if it were to pass, would need tremendous outreach in order to change behavior.

After four years in the House of Representatives, Kagi already knew that tragedy provides an unfortunate cause for legislation; too often it takes a personal story to change the law. She had seen photographs of Maria before the accident, and was struck by the fact that Maria was still a lovely young woman, but not recognizable from the photos. She was obviously still very fragile.

The unsecured load bill was scheduled for a full senate vote on April 14. It had already moved through the house committee chaired by Al O'Brien by a wide margin. Robin and Maria drove down to witness the vote, finding seats in the senate balcony, where not even cushions could keep the wooden benches from becoming unbearably hard. Robin thought that the building seemed cold, as though the granite walls rendered it incapable of absorbing human warmth. Robin was adamant that lawmakers know that she and Maria were watching and listening. They needed to see the possible outcome of driving with an unsecured load. She would not allow what had happened to her daughter to be out of sight or out of mind of the senators.

The scheduled time for the vote came and went. Still, Robin remained in the gallery above the senate floor, afraid that if she left her seat she might miss the vote. An older senator came up from below and walked carefully down to their seats above the railing. "I'm sorry for this delay. We're going to get to your bill as soon as we can," he promised.

It was hard for Maria to sit there for so long; at times she had to rest her head on her mother's lap. Finally, in the late afternoon, their bill was announced. After Luke Esser made a final argument to approve it, the vote began. As each senator's name was called, the response was the same: "Aye!"

Then there was a nay vote. Although it wouldn't affect the final outcome of the bill, the nay was disturbing nonetheless. What possible objection could a senator have to the bill? Representative Kagi was sitting in on the senate vote. Ruth could feel Robin's eyes upon her as she approached the senator who had cast the nay vote. If he had an objection it could put the bill back to committee or cause the bill to die. "Could we step outside for a minute?"

In the hallway outside senate chambers, Ruth asked the senator why he was opposed to the bill.

"I'm concerned about where you intend to draw the line," the senator replied. "Are you trying to say that it would be a crime if I were to lose a teddy bear from the back of my pickup truck?"

Kagi thought about who the senator's constituents were and how they might react to the law. Many of them were ranchers and cowboys, people who worked everyday with pickups and other vehicles, and who wouldn't appreciate being told how to load them. That wasn't an argument that could be settled quickly.

"No," she told him. "The point is to secure objects so they don't cause property damage or physical harm."

He agreed on the spot to vote for the bill if it was amended to include the word "substantial" before injury. It was the difference of one word but it made the vote unanimous and allowed the bill to return to the House for a final vote. Every single senator voted to approve the bill.

The text of House Bill 1478 was divided into seven sections, with the new language:

"A person is guilty of failure to secure a load in the first degree if he or she, with criminal negligence, fails to secure a load, or part of a load to his or her vehicle in compliance with subsection (1),(2), or (3) of this section and causes substantial bodily harm to another.

Failure to secure a load in the first degree is a gross misdemeanor."

The House approved the bill on April 19, 2005. "Maria's Law" was finally on its way to the governor's desk for signing.

The week the bill passed two people died on the Golden Gate Freeway in the Bay Area after a large piece of metal on the roadway struck their vehicle. Robin and Maria learned about the accident from a reporter for the Los Angeles Times, who interviewed Robin and Maria for a story about the dangers of road debris.

The governor signed "Maria's Law" on May 12, 2005. Robin and Maria made the drive to Olympia, but instead of sitting in the gallery they waited in the antechamber of the governor's office, surrounded by oil portraits of every Washington governor since statehood. They had been invited to the ceremonial signing in which the legislative sponsors and the governor all pose for official photos. Accompanying the Abels were Sherry Palmiter and Robin's nephew Kellen. Before the signing, Robin was a little nervous about meeting the governor, Christine Gregoire.

"Come on back," a woman said to Robin and Maria, leading them out of the public space. Suddenly a small elegant woman came towards them.

"I'm Chris Gregoire," she said. "I wanted to have a chance to meet with you."

She led them into a large office and gestured toward two white loveseats. "With a law like this," Gregoire said, "I like to meet with the family beforehand so I can have the opportunity to thank you personally for what you've done."

Afterwards Robin couldn't remember exactly what they discussed, only that Gregoire was so sincere that she felt strangely at ease with her. Maria seemed particularly shy. Robin asked Gregoire about her daughters. Then Gregoire's assistant led them into an adjoining room for the actual signing. Luke Esser and Ruth Kagi were there, along with several of the governor's staff. Robin and Maria stood on either side of the governor as she ceremonially signed the bill for the photographer. Gregoire then presented Robin with the pen she used to sign the new bill. It was only some time later that Robin realized that this was one of the most signifcant days of her life.

"Maria's Law" would go into effect on July 24, 2005.

Robin needed to get busy.

24

With the return of summer, Robin cast around for new activities for Maria. Over the winter Maria had been making jewelry, arranging beads by color and size. Robin arranged for her to sell some of her jewelry at the Renton Farmers Market and she had a banner made: Designs by Maria. Maria was bored with television and movies; besides she only wanted to watch films she'd seen before her accident. Maria seemed depressed. Robin came up with another plan, and this one involved dogs again.

When they had lived in Utah, Maria called her mom one day and said, "I just did something that's going to make you really mad."

"Tell me right now," Robin told her.

"I got a puppy."

"Take it back," Robin said.

"But Mom," Maria said teasingly. "It's a golden." She knew Robin had always wanted a golden retriever.

"I'll take a look," Robin said, as though the outcome wasn't obvious. They named the puppy Beau. He was a year old when they moved back from Utah; Artie, their German pointer, had just passed away.

While Maria was at Harborview, Robin had got permission for Beau to visit on Easter Sunday. Robin couldn't help thinking that Maria's brain injury would vanish like a movie version of amnesia if something could jog her memory back into place. She hoped it would be the golden. When Robin arrived with Beau, Maria didn't respond at all. Then she went into the bathroom and the dog followed, as though aware that she needed careful tending. At the sound of the dog prancing on the linoleum floor Maria burst out, "Sit Beau!" It was her moment of clarity.

After Beau, their next golden retriever had been Jorja. Robin had hoped to breed her but she needed surgery when she was young and couldn't have puppies. Before her accident, when Maria was living in an apartment, she would call home and ask Robin to put Jorja on to "sing" to her. Even after Robin had found the lap dog Sammy for Maria, Robin was still considering a guide dog for Maria, perhaps training their own dog since she didn't qualify through an agency. Robin contacted a breeder about possible goldens. That's when she learned about Sky, a thirteen-month-old female.

Robin took Maria to Tacoma to meet the female golden retriever. The dog bounded through the open door but then instinctively dropped to its belly and crawled the last ten feet to Maria as though sensing her fragility. Sky went home with them that day. Robin held onto the idea of breeding Sky in the future.

Given Maria's love of dogs, in particular her Cavalier, Robin had also been thinking that dog training could be rewarding for both of them. Robin wondered if there were a way for Maria to train Sammy to be her therapy dog. Before the accident both she and Maria had been intrigued with training guide dogs, partly influenced by their across-the-lake neighbors, Howard and his wife Robin, who raised puppies for guiding.

Sammy was completely dedicated to Maria and was so smart that Robin was positive he could do more with training. She called a national organization for therapy dog training and asked for a local referral.

"I need a trainer who can think outside of the box," Robin said.

Robin's referral put her in contact with Diane Rich, a highly experienced dog trainer, and an expert in dog behavior and pet therapy who was already on her way to becoming officially recognized as one of Washington's top ten dog trainers. Diane not only trained dogs, she trained and evaluated trainers. Although Maria's combination of disabilities was a challenge, that wasn't what made working with her unique for Diane. It was the fact that Maria was to be the handler. Normally a therapy dog is trained and then placed with a disabled person. In Maria's case the person with disabilities would also be doing the training. Frankly, Diane loved the challenge and was honored to work with Maria. Maria had her good days and her bad days, but it was nothing Diane couldn't deal with.

When Diane started working with Maria and Sammy at the cabin, Sammy didn't know any commands. One of the biggest problems to overcome was that if Maria gave him the command to "sit," for instance, how would she know if he had responded? Diane had to devise new methods for evaluating follow-through of commands. She also had to assess what specific duties Maria required of Sammy. These duties would include Sammy being able to communicate to Maria when she needed to step down from the deck, or guiding her to the gate beside the driveway. They all worked diligently, once a week in the beginning.

If Sammy was going to become a certified therapy dog he would need a special harness. Maria ordered one, but it would take months for it to be fabricated. Meanwhile Maria and Sammy had to make do with a regular leash. When the harness arrived, it turned out to be way too big for Sammy. Robin regretted the waste of time and money. Looking in the Yellow Pages under horses, Robin called a man named Phil in Kent, an expert in custom leatherwork. He agreed to make a harness for Sammy. Robin and Maria and Sammy drove out to his home. He was a very tall, lanky man. Judging from the way he looked at Maria, Robin was sure he recognized her from the news stories. His eyes filled with tears but he never asked any questions. Instead he led them to the workshop in his barn so that he could measure Sammy.

"Come on little doggie," he said stooping over Sammy and feeling him with his hands. Then he recorded several measurements, including the distance between Maria's hands when her arms were at her side and Sammy's neck. "Okay," he said. "I have enough." He had never made a harness for a guide-dog before. When the harness was done it fit Sammy perfectly. He even added on a pouch for Maria to store small items. Robin always thought of Phil as yet another unexpected angel in their lives.

Of all the activities that Robin devised for Maria as therapies, she still looks back on the dog training as the most successful. Maria applied herself to handling Sammy in a way that Robin hadn't seen since the accident. She didn't know which one of them was going to receive more benefit, the dog or the daughter.

The Maria Federici Foundation was created in the summer of 2005 because of Robin's promise to Norm. A former T-Mobile co-worker, Gary Abrahams, took the lead in filing incorporation documents for the 501(3c) non-profit. The original board members were Robin, Sherry Palmiter, Robert Ott, Carole Kirkpatrick, Dan Pollack, Krysten Cook and Maria's friend, Therese Sangster. Sherry had been helping Robin tirelessly ever since Maria's injury; she took charge of the web site and supporting materials. Although crafting the exact words of their mission statement took time, everyone agreed with their stated goals: *To save lives by educating drivers on the importance of safely securing loads. To encourage lawmakers and enforcement agencies to establish and enforce laws that result in safer roads. To assist and comfort those whose lives are impacted by vehicle-related road debris injuries, or death.*

Just as the Maria Federici Foundation officially launched, Robin received a message on the web site from the Department of Ecology that put their mission into play immediately. It was from Megan Warfield, from Washington State's Department of Ecology, asking how her agency could help. Robin was both surprised and grateful; how often does a government agency contact an individual offering assistance?

The Department of Ecology (DOE) had been the driving force behind the state's previous efforts to educate the public about these matters. In 2002 it had launched a campaign of radio ads, brochures, and billboards with the slogan "Litter and it will hurt," which implied that getting caught littering would hurt a violator's wallet. The message also spoke to aesthetics: littering harms the environment. But the slogan's most literal meaning, that littering could hurt someone physically, didn't occur to many people until they heard about Maria's accident.

Megan's career had always been in litter. For the past ten years she'd served as director of Washington's anti-litter campaign. In her words, she preaches the religion of litter, using every means possible to educate people on the cost of littering, to the environment, to the state, to the individual. Even for Megan, litter doesn't seem like the right word for what gets dropped on and along the roadways. Cigarette butts, fast food wrappers, plastic bags, bottles and beer cans—all are easily labeled litter. But what about toilets, wood pallets, rolls of insulation, tables, chairs, and ladders? You name it—it's probably fallen on a roadway.

Before the state launched its campaign in 2002, the Department of Ecology conducted research to determine what measures would be most effective in changing people's habits.

First they interviewed citizens about their habits and reasons for littering. Essentially the answer was laziness, coupled with the unlikelihood of any financial consequences. In the second phase researchers actually conducted litter surveys along various roadways, sorting it into categories based on where it was collected and what it was.

Based on this research, the DOE prepared a multi-agency launch of a new educational campaign called "Litter and It Will Hurt." It emphasized that people caught littering on the road would be fined, and that the State Patrol would be on the lookout for violators. Television commercials and radio announcements were made. Litter bags and posters were distributed. A web site was created and a telephone hotline was set up for people to call if they witnessed someone littering. In response to hotline calls, the DOE mailed stern letters to the registered owners of vehicles letting them know that littering was an infraction subject to a penalty. The DOE also produced an annoying jingle that Megan feels she will be lucky to outlive.

Megan and her staff quickly realized that the campaign was successful. Each year, the number of calls to the hotline climbed by the thousands. In its best year, 17,000 calls were made to the hotline and 17,000 letters were sent out to households. When Megan's department did follow-up surveys, ninety-two percent of those who'd received a letter said they would not litter again.

The DOE's field research had shown that the majority of litter wasn't being thrown out of windows, it was escaping from trucks and trailers whose loads weren't properly covered or secured. But even the State Patrol wasn't tracking a connection between road debris and road safety. Megan applied for grants so that the State Patrol could do what are called "emphasis patrols," where officers specifically look for litter law violators. But these were ineffective because tickets could not be issued unless an officer actually witnessed the violation.

Then Maria's accident happened. "Litter and it will hurt" took on a completely different meaning. When Megan first spoke to Robin she offered her view as a safety professional. "An accident is usually something that couldn't have been prevented," she told her. "An incident is something that could have been prevented. What happened to your daughter could have been prevented." Robin understood the difference immediately.

Megan had closely followed the progress of the new unsecured load law as it worked through the legislative process; her agency had submitted statistical data and a letter of support. She was thrilled when "Maria's Law" was enacted. Not only would the Department of Ecology provide program support, it would work with the Washington State Department of Transportation, the Washington State Patrol, and every county in the state to promote enforcement. When Megan got in touch with Robin, she had access to resources from the State's Litter Fund, and a grant to produce brochures and an educational video about securing a load properly. Within a month of the first conversation with Megan, Robin and Maria were participating in a video that featured Maria's story and spelled out the new law and its consequences.

The same month that "Maria's Law" took effect, Reader's Digest published a story called *Danger on the Road: Stray animals, falling trees, flying debris. Why hidden hazards are a rising threat – and how to steer clear.* The article mentioned the death of the celebrated film director, Alan Pakula, when a metal pipe that had fallen from a vehicle pierced his car's windshield and speared him in the head. Robin was interviewed for the story, which reported that "1.6 million car accidents per year involve trees, animals and road debris. . ."

Fatalities due to road debris were on the rise, according to the story, going from 298 deaths in 1999 to 427 in 2003.

Since auto accidents are often improperly coded, the numbers were probably far too low, the writer reported. The article made the important point that incidents such as those that killed Pakula and severely injured Maria are frequently written off as "freak accidents."

Traffic safety numbers vary between agencies, with a study commissioned by the Automobile Association of America (AAA) attributing 25,000 accidents per year to vehicular road debris. To Robin that number screamed "frequent accidents" rather than "freak accidents." Plus she had learned to think of them as incidents, not accidents; they could have been prevented. The numbers will always vary between studies, depending on tracking methods. An accident's root cause isn't always known or tracked the same way by different agencies. If a driver veers off the road because of debris, does the debris get classified as the cause?

All the accident tracking agencies posed the question of where road debris comes from. The study conducted for the AAA Foundation in 2004 identified commercial truckers as the top violators for unsecured loads and the dominant source of road debris, mostly due to blown tires. But Robin, after studying the issue at length, began to believe that the average citizen was the source of most of the road debris that caused accidents.

At first, Robin felt overwhelmed by all the data. Should she start by trying to reach commercial truckers or people cleaning out their garages? Should she target employers or citizens on their way to the dump? How could she, as just one person, make the biggest impact? The president of AAA's national organization, Peter Kissinger, who was well aware of Maria's road debris incident, encouraged her to tell her personal story to as many drivers as possible. She decided to start locally by contacting all the occupational safety organizations in the state. The first listing under "safety" in the Yellow Pages was Argus Pacific–specialists in workplace safety.

The man who picked up the phone when Robin called Argus Pacific was Ray Clouatre. If you included his work in the Air Force, which Clouatre usually did, one could say he had been working in the safety field all of his adult life. In the military he'd specialized in bomb disposal, but was also trained in security, firefighting, and emergency medicine. After being discharged from the military, he spent eight years working for the Evergreen Safety Council, a private, nonprofit company that teaches safety training to businesses, governmental entities, and communities in the Pacific Northwest.

All that Robin had at that point was sheer desire to educate "John Q. Public." She didn't have any literature or posters, just the power of what her family had experienced. Clouatre realized that she really needed to speak with someone at Evergreen because its mission was public safety. Robin's message matched Evergreen's goals and its focus on outreach. But Clouatre said he had plenty of contacts within the safety industry whom he was willing to email on her behalf.

"Do you know about the Governor's Safety Conference?" he asked Robin.

Robin didn't, but she was keenly interested. Clouatre had been involved with the annual fall conference as a volunteer and presenter for years, and thought Robin's efforts to promote the new unsecured load law would be a natural fit. The conference, which attracted around 3,000 workplace safety and health professionals each year, was a joint venture between Washington's Department of Labor and Industry and the Washington Governor's Industrial Health and Safety Board. Char Alexander from Labor and Industry was the conference manager. Clouatre gave Robin her contact information.

Robin called Alexander, who agreed with Clouatre that she'd be perfect for the conference. When Robin told her she couldn't afford the significant fee for having a booth, Alexander told her not to worry: she'd find a sponsor for her.

The Tacoma Convention Center was packed with booths, mostly staffed by vendors with products to sell. Robin sat in an empty booth, behind an almost bare table, with only a few brochures to offer. Attendees would usually glance at displays to see if there were any freebies. To most of them, Robin looked like she might just be resting in an unoccupied space. Then something happened. She began to attract a lot of people to her table. Robin later told Clouatre that, frustrated by peoples' lack of interest she finally started calling out to them: "Don't you want to know why I'm here?"

Once she got people to talk with her they were spellbound. Many had heard about Maria and wanted to know how she was faring. People told Robin their own stories about damage or near-misses on the roads caused by debris. Word about her presence seemed to spread throughout the convention center and attendees flocked to her. She made contact with organizations that wanted her to speak with their employees.

That was Robin's first appearance at the Governor's Safety Conference, in 2005, She has attended every conference since then, but the one that gives Clouatre his greatest sense of pride was one in Spokane when Robin and Maria were introduced at the conference luncheon. By then almost everyone in the safety industry had heard Maria Federici's story, and used it in their work to stress the importance of load safety. Hundreds of people jumped to their feet to give them a standing ovation.

Clouatre had given Robin the name of the new director at the Evergreen Safety Council, and she did a little research on the outfit before giving Tom Odegaard a call. The average person might not realize that traffic flaggers have to be officially trained and certified. Their training is just one of hundreds of programs offered through the American Association of Safety

Councils. The Evergreen Safety Council is a founding member of the national group and has been providing programs in Washington for seventy-five years.

Odegaard's resume included a stint working on natural gas pipeline safety, including the public education program, "Call Before You Dig," which informed homeowners and businesses of the need to check with gas companies before digging into soil where gas lines might lie. He had heard about Maria Federici, but hadn't connected the incident to his current focus at the Council of teaching defensive driver training. When they spoke on the phone, the traffic safety aspect of her story clicked for him immediately, especially because workplace safety could involve being the one to lose a load or the one affected by road debris while driving. Odegaard invited her to address a Traffic Safety Conference that fall.

Robin's message in front of the traffic safety folks really struck a nerve, and Odegaard could see that her story needed a wider audience. He gave her more contacts in the safety field, such as the Traffic Safety Commission, and the Department of Labor and Industries in Olympia.

Odegaard appreciated Robin's energy and purpose, and he felt good opening doors for her. Odegaard was able to make sure the "Secure Your Load" video was available on the Evergreen Safety Council website for free downloading. As a member of the American Association of Safety Councils, Evergreen Safety Council was able to connect with the National Safety Council. At the very least, the Evergreen Safety Council reaches up to 3,500 businesses a month with its newsletter–access to the national organizations made its reach even broader.

After "Maria's Law" officially went into effect, Megan Warfield retooled the Department of Ecology's litter program to focus on larger debris, with an emphasis on Maria's personal story. It was the turning point in the Department of Ecology's campaign. After that time, virtually every person Megan talked to about the "Secure Your Load" program already knew what had happened to Maria. When Megan did training with the Washington State Patrol, she noticed they felt a new responsibility for enforcing the law. State Patrol officers often stayed in contact with Megan after their training, sending her photos of what they'd seen on the roadway and letting her know about other accidents that might not have been officially linked to road debris.

When the DOE received word that some citizens were confused by the logistics of securing their load, the Department of Ecology created another brochure entitled "Tips on Securing Your Load." DOE also produced a second video on the topic, this one geared to law enforcement professionals.

Unfortunately, Megan never lacked for people with firsthand experience to talk about the perils of road debris as she took the campaign around the state: the family of a man who died because of an escaped tarp; a man killed in Tacoma avoiding a mattress; a woman injured as she veered around a dining table in her lane at dusk.

Yet Megan's work, though aimed at saving money and saving lives, is constantly threatened by budget cuts. In her mind no one really knows the full costs of litter to society. No one is tracking close calls or unreported lost objects, the dented cars, broken windshields, and accidents caused by such objects as tools, buckets, tires, toilets, and ladders.

Megan could understand completely that Maria might want to try to forget about the accident and go on with her life. But what happened to her had taken on a life of its own. Maria's high profile story had surely prevented other accidents from happening in a way that mere fines could not. Perhaps the only people, after all, who know the full costs of road litter were people such as Robin and Maria.

CHAPTER
25

Before her birthday in December, Robin wrote a wish list. Item number one was to be able to get access to the people who used transfer stations in King County. It was the largest county in the state, with nine transfer stations. Robin had identified that residents and contractors trucking debris to transfer stations were extremely likely to have unsafe loads. They had garage cleanouts and old barbeque grills, broken wheelbarrows and ladders tossed on top of yard waste. Robin figured that if she could get to King County, then other counties in the state would follow suit. She wanted to work with King County's Public Works Department and Solid Waste Division. So getting a contact there was high on the wish list she took with her to a meeting with Norm Maleng–he knew all the King County managers. Her brother Bobby had sent Maleng an email to warn him that it was Robin's birthday, and she had a list of action items. Norm had already set the wheels in motion, working directly with King County Executive Ron Sims to determine how the county could best support the new law.

As for Maria, she received an unexpected and seemingly magical gift for her second Christmas after the accident. She was given a prosthetic right eye to go along with her remaining, though sightless, left eye. The ocular specialists had created a sort of over-size contact lens that went over Maria's left eye, which was shrinking away and would also need replacing later.

The prosthetic eye had a type of shelf that allowed Maria's eyelids to stay open. The first eye had a beautiful brown color, so similar to the eye color that Maria was born with that Robin realized how much she had always identified her daughter by her chocolate eyes and exquisite eyebrows. "Maria has a beautiful, brown eye!" Robin heralded.

Early in 2006 it occurred to Robin that with all the specialized work on Maria's face, no one seemed to be evaluating her neurological progress. The only neurologist on Robin's list of Maria's doctors to call was Dr. Copass.

Robin had heard that when Copass started at Harborview he was hired to work in the Emergency Department, not Neurology. Copass never left Emergency Services, although he did continue to see some neurology patients in clinic. When Robin called his office she was informed that he wasn't accepting new neurology patients. "Just give him my daughter's name," Robin told the receptionist. His office called back the next day to schedule an appointment. Robin knew that Copass wouldn't be able to resist treating Maria. He was the one who had pronounced what had happened to Maria as "beyond catastrophic."

Robin had seen Copass with medical students at Harborview. She knew he could be formidable, but when Robin and Maria first went to see him at his clinic, tears welled up in his eyes as he gazed upon Maria's face.

"You will always be Dr. Hopper's finest work," he said. "Maria, you are his Mona Lisa."

Hearing those words from Copass was a gift, as was his assessment of Robin's therapeutic care of Maria.

"Superb," he later pronounced – under oath. By asking Maria seeming simple questions and running a feather along each side of her face, he provided Robin with an instant feedback. Maria didn't have any feeling on the left side of her face, and no muscle response. But her mental acuity had improved. Robin realized that she was the one who most needed Copass–otherwise she had no sense of whether she was on the right path with Maria's therapy.

A major incentive for Robin to work on changing the law regarding unsecured loads was the fact that Maria didn't qualify for crime victim compensation. Under the old law, what had happened to her wasn't considered a crime. But there was still one problem with "Maria's Law." It didn't specify that someone injured as a result of an unsecured load would be eligible for the Crime Victims Compensation Fund. Governor Gregoire was the one who noticed the oversight. Representative Kagi assured Robin that she would introduce an amendment to the law at the beginning of the next session. But she warned Robin that it would have fiscal impact, meaning that the legislature would need to consider the financial implications for the state budget of adding another eligible crime to the Crime Victims Compensation Program. Bills with fiscal impact can be more challenging to pass, but there was obviously strong support for "Maria's Law" based on the previous votes in the House and Senate. On the bright side, Robin already had a much better sense of navigating the legislature.

Depending on her mood, Robin would think, I'm just a mom, I can't do this alone. At other times she felt that mothers were capable of superhuman strength when it came to protecting their children, and she was astounded by what she could accomplish on sheer adrenalin. She continued to use the phrase, "Never underestimate the power of a pissed-off mom," which became a sort of mantra for her. Robin still didn't know what her next move would be, but she knew she needed to keep going forward. If she could get one bill passed, she could get a second in another state, and someday perhaps even a national law.

On January 11, Kagi introduced the bill to amend "Maria's Law" so that it would link to Crime Victims Compensation. Less than two weeks later, a man named Sandy Harmon died in Tacoma, Washington, when his car was crushed by other cars that were swerving to avoid a large tarp that had fallen off a semi-truck. "My son is gone for somebody's negligence," said his mother, Laraine Harmon. A few weeks after that fatality, Elizabeth Chaffin and her niece were nearly killed on the Olympic Peninsula when a piece of plywood flew off a vehicle's load and crashed through their windshield. To support the amendment to "Maria's Law," Robin and Maria were again making frequent trips to Olympia. Robin testified at the public hearing along with representatives from Labor and Industry and the Crime Victims Compensation Program. Since the first bill had already established the crime, the focus in this legislative session was on why the victims of this crime should be eligible for compensation. A summary of the bill stated, "Victims of this crime shouldn't have to suffer. Assistance should be provided for them. Crime Victims Compensation is already available for the victims of other vehicular crimes, such as negligent vehicular homicide and driving under the influence."

Ruth Kagi left a shocking voicemail for Robin near the end of the 2006 legislative session. "The bill died in committee, but I would be happy to reintroduce it next year," she said. Robin felt physically ill. She had just turned on KOMO-TV News to see if there was any word about the bill. As she thought about Ruth's message, news anchor Kathi Goertzen reported that a drunk driving bill had died in committee that day. Robin emailed Goertzen while she was still broadcasting live that her bill had died as well. A few minutes later, Robin received an instant message from Goertzen on her computer. "Well that really pisses me off," she wrote.

Robin had met Goertzen several times since Maria's accident. She had interviewed Maria after she got her new eyes. Goertzen was involved in a golden retrievers rescue group, finding good homes for dogs that owners no longer wanted. She and Robin had bonded over Robin's golden retrievers, and Robin trusted her implicitly.

Immediately after Robin informed her that her bill had "died," Goertzen contacted KOMO's Olympia reporter, Keith Eldridge, and asked him to find out why. "So I went to work to find out what happened," Eldridge said later. "At our request, the bill's sponsor, Representative Ruth Kagi, checked to see if the bill should have been exempt from the cut-off since it was tied to the state budget. It turns it out it was still eligible to be voted on."

Early the next morning Robin emailed Norm's Chief of Staff, Dan Satterberg, with the message, "Remember when you said to contact you when I needed help? Well, we are in the home stretch on this legislation and I really need your help."

Satterberg dispatched his colleague, Tom McBride, to Olympia. In the face of media scrutiny and support from the Prosecutor's Office, the amendment to Maria's law came alive again. Within twenty-four hours of being pronounced dead, the bill was not only revived, but passed unanimously in committee in the final hours.

Acknowledging KOMO-TV's role in saving the bill, Robin said on camera, "By shining a light on it, you at KOMO-4 really made a huge difference–just asking pointed questions of the right people."

Even Governor Gregoire, in a meeting with the press on the day of the signing, cited KOMO's role. "I thank you [KOMO-TV] for making sure it was brought to the legislature's attention," Gregoire said. "It was a fast and furious fifty-nine days and things were lost. This didn't have a right to be lost. So thanks, this was the right thing to do."

When Robin and Maria were invited back to meet privately once again with Chris Gregoire, before the signing ceremony for the amendment to Maria's Law, Gregoire greeted Robin and Maria by saying, "It's good to have you back." At the signing, Kagi remarked to the Governor, "If you knew what she'd done to get this bill passed, you'd be calling it 'Robin's Law.'"

CHAPTER

26

King County Executive Ron Sims felt like Maria's accident had happened in "his backyard." He didn't need extra coaxing to issue a mandate to his division managers to identify ways to prevent an incident like this from happening again.

It was obvious the Solid Waste Division would play the lead role. This group maintains the county's nine transfer stations, which are the number-one destination for household and commercial debris. As part of her broad job description Polly Young was in charge of communicating waste disposal guidelines to all households, and training transfer station scale operators who deal with the public as well as garbage handlers, contractors, and landscapers. Young needed to figure out a way to educate all these groups about Maria's Law. Working with Polly Young was on Robin's wish list.

For nearly twenty years, signs outside the transfer stations had reminded all users to cover their loads. Since 1994, the scale operators, who calculate dump fees for each vehicle, had been told to add a small penalty fee if a vehicle's load was unsecured. The surcharge wasn't designed to create revenue but to change behavior. These fees were designated to fund additional educational efforts. But the scale operators were loathe to tack on the fee because it angered the public. Young struggled for years to get the scale operators to apply the surcharge, but few ever did.

Young believed Robin could help with the problem. In February of 2006, during an annual training program for scale operators, Polly introduced Robin as a guest speaker. Most of the operators had never heard of her before. Then Robin began, "I've had firsthand experience with an unsecured load. . . ."

As she told the story about Maria, the room fell completely silent. By the end, many people had tears in their eyes, including Young. After Robin's talk, scale operators were able to make a connection between the unsecured load fee and a human being. Immediately afterwards, the collection rate for the unsecured load surcharge quadrupled.

Transfer stations, however, were just part of the picture. Polly Young also studied how to build public awareness about load safety and how to create an enforcement campaign. Solid Waste sent letters to every household and business account. The division contacted large corporate users such as Boeing and many municipalities. The King County Executive issued a directive to all King County employees mandating that they secure their loads. Meanwhile, Young began working with other agencies, such as the Department of Ecology, safety organizations, and other counties. And she continued working with Robin. Using a variety of grants and limited budgets, Young and Robin collaborated on brochures and videos, downloadable resources, and a website, all while planning a giant "kick-off" event at Qwest Field, slated for April 2006.

Polly tracked the data religiously: the spike in transfer station fees after Robin spoke to the scale operators, the number of hotline phone calls to report unsecured loads, the increase in citations since the Washington State Patrol began targeting load violators near King County transfer stations. By all accounts, more and more people were getting the message about the need to secure their loads.

John Carlson was driving on the freeway when the sixteen-wheeler ahead of him hit a huge chunk of wood and sent it airborne. He didn't have time to duck; he didn't even have time to swerve. The wood hit the hood of his car and then cracked the windshield without penetrating the glass. Carlson was lucky that day because otherwise the headlines might have read, "Construction Safety Director Killed by Construction Debris."

Carlson's field of safety expertise is the construction industry. Robin had cold-called him when he was Safety Director for the Association of General Contractors (AGC), Washington's largest trade association and an affiliate of the largest construction industry association in the United States. Perhaps because of his own run-in with road debris, he was immediately willing to do what Robin asked: get word to the general public that loads needed to be secured. Carlson has daughters about the same age as Maria; he knew about her accident from media reports. His first instinct was to meet Robin in person, so he drove out to the cabin and spent several hours with Robin and Maria.

Carlson has seen serious accidents firsthand, having worked on incidents over the years that involved four fatalities and seventeen serious injuries. Still, seeing what had happened to Maria was traumatic for him. After spending a little time with them, he began to enjoy their mother-daughter dynamics. Robin was impassioned and tenacious, bubbling with ideas for how to get the message about Maria's Law to various industries and the general public. Maria was blunt and extremely witty. She made him laugh, but stated clearly that she wanted to get on with her life and that the public outreach was her mom's thing. He set Robin up with quite a few professional contacts.

After meeting Maria, Carlson would sometimes begin the safety classes he teaches by asking a question: "How many of you woke up this morning and thought, today would be a good day to die or to kill someone?" He wanted to get their attention, to make them realize that little things can mean the difference between life and death. In his mind, if someone didn't take the extra time to secure a load, they were just lazy. But if they could learn that laziness can kill, he believed they would make the right choice.

Rick Gleason met Robin when she had a booth at the 2006 Governor's Safety Conference in Spokane. He was up to speed on "Maria's Law" and how it was now attached to the Crime Victims Compensation Fund. Gleason's work in Occupational Health and Safety dovetailed closely with Labor and Industry, which administered the Crime Victims Compensation Fund. Robin's focus on road safety spoke to him because he was obsessed by the fact that the number one cause of death for workers in the United States is motor vehicle accidents while on the job. There were 5,700 such deaths in 2008, and that doesn't include workers who were on their way to or from work.

When it came time for Gleason to find a speaker for what was then the Puget Sound Safety Summit, a monthly meeting of safety professionals, he thought of Robin. He had a small budget for an honorarium but Robin didn't even ask for a fee. "At least let us pay you mileage," he told her.

The Safety Summit folks had no idea what was coming the morning Gleason introduced Robin solely by name, letting her story provide the context. Most speakers usually discussed topics such as how to comply with the latest Occupational Health and Safety rules on heat stress or welding; Robin spoke from the heart. Rick still remembers the two sentences that gave him chills: "I can't tell you how to secure your load. All I can tell you is to secure the load as though your son or daughter were driving behind you."

Ron Sims had been on the King County Council since 1985, so when he became King County Executive in 1997 his working relationship with Norm Maleng was already long-established. But the connection went beyond their roles as the highest elected officials in King County Government–they had a spiritual bond too. Sims was an ordained Baptist minister and Maleng was an Episcopal lay eucharistic minister. Although their party affiliations were different, the men's mutual dedication to their work and one another was the same.

As King County Executive, Sims was the person at the top of the masthead, ultimately in charge of all the departments in county government, including Harborview, the Courthouse, King County Council, public transportation, transfer stations, landfills, the jail, hazardous waste collection, many parks, and of course the Prosecutor's Office.

When Maleng asked Sims to send off a letter of support for "Maria's Law," Sims was proud of Maleng's office for its role in drafting such common-sense legislation. How could anyone oppose it, he wondered? Sims didn't think citizens were being malicious when they failed to secure things in the backs of their trucks, just lazy or ignorant of the danger. "In a million years you could never make up for the harm if something happened," he said. "Never in a million years." Sims ordered all county employees who carried loads to be trained in how to secure them properly.

The "Secure Your Load" kick-off event was at Qwest Field, the Seattle Seahawks' stadium, on April 13, 2006–and it was a big deal. Sims was proud of the County's initiative in planning the event because it included so many different agencies and departments. The county's Solid Waste Division had teamed up with the State Department of Transportation, the Washington State Patrol, and the Evergreen Safety Council. Within King

County, the Prosecutor himself and his staff were involved, along with Public Works and Community Relations people.

Not until the day of the event did Sims get a chance to meet Maria or her mother. Although Sims had ministered for his church in some grim situations, he didn't realize the full dimension of Maria's tragedy until he stood beside her in person. He had felt badly for Maria and her family when he'd first heard about the accident, and had done everything he could as King County Executive to promote "Maria's Law" and to educate the public about it. But when this small, sweet-voiced young woman stood at his side, it really shook him.

On that breezy April day at Qwest Field, Maria stood between Sims and Maleng. Her mother was nearby. As a father, Sims wished she had not had to go through all her suffering, that he could somehow turn back the clock so that Maria was on that road ten minutes earlier or ten minutes later. He wished that the laws could have protected her better. Channeling his emotions, Sims simply kissed Maria on the forehead before collecting himself to speak.

The event at Qwest Field accomplished all the things that each participant desired because they all had the same mission: saving lives, reducing litter, and giving people a reason to change their behavior when driving with a load. Speakers and demonstrations emphasized various elements of the new law, how it would be enforced, and its anticipated impact. It was also a day to celebrate the law and that its public awareness was already climbing. A Parks Department employee demonstrated the proper techniques for securing a load. Banners and brochures with links to the website were distributed, along with videos made by the Department of Ecology and the Washington State Patrol. The event addressed Robin's greatest concerns about how people would translate the law into action. Securing a load didn't mean that it was below the sides of the tailgate, or that it was so heavy it wouldn't fly out, or so light that it wouldn't hurt anyone.

Securely means safely, and fastened means to tie down so that the load won't budge. For a load to be "securely fastened," whether it is heavy or light, it must be restrained so that it doesn't budge or shift if the driver needs to speed up or brake. It is for the situation that a driver doesn't, or can't anticipate.

During the previous months Maria hadn't wanted to accompany Robin on any speaking engagements. She certainly hadn't wanted her picture posted at any "garbage dumps," as she called them, and Robin had respected her wishes. But Maria didn't need to be coaxed to attend the event at Qwest Field; she asked to attend. Robin assured her that she didn't need to speak unless she chose to do so. Perhaps Maria would gain a sense of what they'd accomplished. Robin was scared but excited about the prospect of reaching so many people, both at the event itself and through the media that would cover it.

A photographer from King County documented the day, in addition to all of the local newspapers and television stations. The most striking photos showed Sims and Maleng standing beside Maria like two devoted uncles.

At one point, Sims asked Robin, "Do you think Maria would be willing to say a few words?"

Robin could tell that Maria felt safe with him. He had been talking to her and Robin had seen her smile at his comments. Robin told him, "Why don't you ask her?"

She didn't take long to agree. Placed in front of a microphone, Maria had a soft but strong voice. She said what she'd often heard her mother say to people. "It doesn't take much more time or much more money [to secure a load]," she said, "just a little more compassion."

All Western Washington media reported on the Qwest event. When Maria heard herself on KIRO-TV she told Robin, "I sound pretty good." Robin could tell she felt a bit like a star. The best of the coverage highlighted the reason for the law and how it would be enforced. One or two reported on another news item that should have been incidental to the safety message. One week earlier attorneys on behalf of Maria had filed a product liability lawsuit in King County Superior Court against U-Haul International, Capron Holdings (the commissioned agent that rented the trailer), and against the driver of the vehicle that lost its load, James Hefley. The timing was unfortunate, because nothing should have distracted from the day's real message: *Secure Your Load.*

Robin preferred The Seattle Times report that stated, in part, that "the 26-year old Renton woman and her mother have attracted powerful allies." Robin smiled when she read that, but the truth was that ever since Maria's accident she'd seen so much good from so many people. Her "powerful allies" were heroes like Norm Maleng who wanted to build a more just world. "Justice has many forms," he had said. While Robin hoped that justice would prevail in the King County Superior Court as well, she felt that giving her and Maria a voice at the Qwest Field event was already a form of justice.

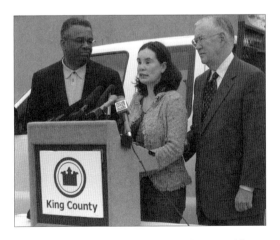

Ron Sims, Maria and Norm Maleng at Qwest Field event
Photo courtesy of King County Department of Natural Resources & Parks

27

Milo Pipkin heard Robin at an Evergreen Safety Council event while he was a safety officer for Waste Management Inc., one of the largest waste and environmental service companies in North America. His first thought was, what if something came loose from one of Waste Management's hundreds of trucks? He wanted every Waste Management driver to hear Robin and Maria's story.

In helping Robin take her story to Waste Management drivers, Pipkin became a driver himself–for Robin and Maria. He would pick Robin and Maria up at their cabin, starting out from his home at 4:00 a.m. Within a matter of months Robin and Maria gave half a dozen talks to drivers in several Waste Management locations in Western Washington. Robin would tell the story about what happened to Maria, show the "Secure Your Load" video, then introduce Maria. Often Maria would just tell stories about Sammy and how important he was to her as a therapy dog. Milo and Robin teased her about whether she was nervous at speaking engagements.

"Why would I be nervous?" she replied. "I can't see anyone."

Pipkin did something once that made Robin terribly upset. It had snowed, and to keep his truck from fishtailing he had put firewood in the back to weigh down the rear wheels. When Robin saw the loose wood, "she had a fit." She reminded him that just because an object is heavy doesn't mean it is secured.

Robin told Pipkin: "Weight is not a form of securement."

He knew she was right. If he'd been going to the transfer station he would have known to secure his load, but he had only been thinking about traction in the snow. Pipkin apologized and bought a cargo net. But it was a reminder that everyone can make mistakes, even someone trained in safety.

Robin returned to her longtime dream of breeding one of her golden retrievers; Jorja hadn't been able to have puppies because of a health problem. Robin began the long process necessary to breed Sky, the female golden they'd acquired as a thirteen-month old. The dog had to pass medical tests and then win an international conformation title. Robin had realized that aside from music and shopping, Maria was most engaged with dogs. "I'm not getting up with the puppies," Maria claimed.

Sky's litter was due within a day of a speech Robin was scheduled to deliver in Leavenworth to the Washington Traffic Safety Commission. "The only reason I might cancel is if my dog has puppies," Robin warned her public health contact,

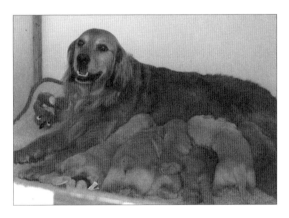

Sky's newborn puppies

Tony Gomez. Sky's breeder came to stay with Robin and Maria as Sky showed signs of labor. The first puppy, "Ben," was born while Robin was in the shower that morning. Jean said she would be able to stay and deliver the puppies so she urged Robin to go ahead and make the trip to Leavenworth. When Robin was introduced she announced that she was up to four puppies; by the time the meeting ended there were six puppies in all. The following days went exactly as Robin had hoped; Maria could not resist the whimpers in the night when a puppy was separated from its mother. She would make her way to the box on the floor, locate the warm puppy, and put it back with its mother. She grew to recognize each one by sound and feel. Ben was the only puppy they kept.

After working with Maria and Sammy for nearly two years, Diane Rich, the dog trainer, thought they were ready for certification as handler and therapy dog. During the second year of their training, Maria, Sammy, Maria's caregiver, and Diane had seemingly gone everywhere together. In order to pass the test, Sammy needed to be able to fulfill his duties no matter what the situation. They had been to malls, schools, Home Depot, nursing homes.

The test would be difficult, but Rich felt confident that Maria and Sammy would succeed. Each requirement of the test would be scored for both dog and handler, either zero points for failure, one point for adequate mastery, or two points for outstanding. Human and dog would be graded together in every category, with the lower score prevailing; if the handler got a one and the dog a two, it would be scored as a one.

Nobody expected Maria and Sammy to do as well as they did: they received perfect scores for every requirement. In all her years as a therapy dog trainer and evaluator, Diane couldn't recall another perfect score. Yet here were Maria and Sammy–a disabled woman who was acting as her own therapy dog's trainer. They had been magnificent and Diane was very proud.

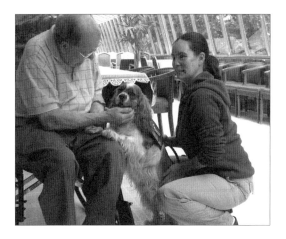

Maria and Sammy in therapy dog training
Photo courtesy of Diane Rich Dog Training, LLC

Robin had found that speaking to one group usually led to opportunities with other groups. Her schedule was becoming so full that she started charging an honorarium to cover her time and travel expenses.

When she talked to contractors or Washington State Ferry Workers, she would think about all those "powerful allies" she had who could open doors for her. It was wonderful to have access to the King County Prosecutor and the Chief of Washington State Patrol, but on any given day she could also call upon those she considered her fellow foot soldiers: Megan Warfield and Polly Young, Tom Odegaard and Milo Pipkin, John Carlson, Ray Clouatre, and Rick Gleason.

The Crime Victim portion of "Maria's Law" went into effect on June 27, 2006. Ten days later a Sheriff's Deputy in Anaheim, California, died following a collision as a result of a stove that had fallen onto the roadway. Tragic incidents had a terrible way of punctuating important milestones in Robin's campaign. But the accident that happened the following month in Seattle would prove to be a milestone in itself: the first application of Maria's Law.

The Coffee family was planning one final camping trip for the end of summer vacation. Gavin Coffee had taken Friday off from work so they could get an early start. His wife Heidi was returning from a church retreat with a van full of teenage girls, including their two daughters. The two younger sons were at the last day of a weeklong soccer camp that always ended with an exhibition scrimmage. The camping gear was ready to be loaded into the van; they had reservations at a campground.

Gavin drove to his Seattle office to check on a work detail before going to pick up the boys at soccer camp. He took I-5 northbound, and was a mile south of his exit at Northeast 175th, speaking by cell phone with his church pastor. What happened next became Washington State Patrol Criminal Investigation Unit Case No. 06-0008878, a multiple car fatality collision/loss of load investigation. Two men, a grandfather and grandson, were driving a pickup truck on I-5, traveling from Queen Anne to Lake Forest Park with various items in the truck bed, including a metal shelving unit that was five-feet long and three-feet wide. Because the shelving was so long, they'd rested one end on the tail gate. There were tie down hooks in the truck bed, but the men hadn't used them; they would regret that choice for the rest of their lives.

As they approached their exit, the shelving unit flew out of the truck. The woman in the car behind them swerved to avoid the object and then lost control, moving left across two lanes of traffic. Her car collided with Gavin's car; he reacted by steering hard to the left but also lost control. Gavin's car, a Honda, was then hit broadside on the driver's side by a Lincoln Town car, and slammed into the freeway barrier. The Lincoln was then struck by a Toyota Camry. The pickup truck continued–its occupants ignorant of what was happening in their wake.

On the other end of Gavin's cell phone call, his pastor heard one exclamation from him, probably when Gavin saw the shelving fall from the truck or when the first car swerved. Then Gavin dropped the phone as he fought to control the car. The pastor heard enough to realize Gavin had been in an accident and probably hadn't survived. Despite people who stopped to help him, and the first responders' efforts, he was pronounced dead at the scene.

Heidi Coffee's nightmare began within minutes. Their pastor called her to say that Gavin had been in an accident and that it sounded very serious. He told her to meet him at Harborview, where he was expected to be sent. A friend took care of the teenage girls while another drove Heidi to the hospital. Heidi and her pastor searched for Gavin but there was no record of him at Harborview. He had not been admitted to Emergency Services. They called other hospitals and still couldn't find him. Finally they went to the accident scene on I-5. They were told by an officer that the driver of the Honda had not survived and had been picked up by the Medical Examiner to take him to the morgue.

When she finally got a call from the Medical Examiner's office, it was to tell her where she could pick up Gavin's personal effects. Heidi didn't get to see Gavin until after the autopsy, which found that the primary cause of death was a crushed neck. His death was later classified as a crime because the second phase of Maria's law had gone into effect seven weeks earlier. Like Maria's accident, Gavin Coffee's occurred within a mile of his home. Out of forty-nine legislative districts in the state, his death was in Representative Ruth Kagi's district.

The two men who lost their load that day were not aware of it until notified by a witness who followed them from the freeway. The grandson drove south past the accident scene to see if it could be true and then went to his grandfather's house nearby. Within the hour the grandfather phoned 9-1-1 to report that he had lost the load that caused the collision on I-5. Washington State Patrol sergeants went to the grandfather's home and spoke to him, learning that the grandson had actually been driving. Both admitted they had been in a hurry because the grandfather's wife had had a doctor's appointment, and they hadn't taken the time to tie down the load. The metal shelving unit was on its way to a garbage dump.

The grandfather and grandson were exactly the kind of people who had no intention of doing harm to anyone and would have given nearly anything to turn back the clock and secure their load. On September 19, 2006, the King County Prosecutor's Office announced its decision to charge both men with criminal negligence in the first degree by failing to secure their load.

"When we lobbied for this law, it was our hope that we would never have to use it," Norm Maleng said in his press release.

Heidi was surprised at all the media interest in Gavin's death. She was wrapped up in planning the funeral, preparing to get four children back to school in a few weeks, and thinking about the fifth child on the way. Heidi and Robin met that fall. Heidi's thirteen-year old daughter, Laurisa, was doing a school project on community involvement and wanted to learn more about the "Secure Your Load" campaign. Laurisa's theme was the fact that every action affects someone else. Heidi and her daughters drove out to Lake Kathleen to meet Robin and Maria. Later, when Laurisa presented her project to her class, she didn't talk about her father's death; she talked about Maria Federici and how her miraculous survival was being used to protect others in the community.

Heidi and Robin met again when Norm Maleng invited them both to his office for their input on sentencing recommendations for the grandfather and grandson. Heidi was struck by how Maleng's staff was clearly devoted to him. But she didn't think he really believed the law would never need to be applied. Heidi considered that a wishful hope, not a realistic one.

Silas Gavin Coffee was six weeks old on January 20, 2007– the day of sentencing at King County District Court for the two men charged in his father's death. Robin and Maria were in the courtroom, Maria's little dog in her lap. Norm's Chief of Staff, Dan Satterberg, was sitting next to Maria. The sentencing was emotional for everyone. Heidi and her brother-in-law both addressed the defendants, telling them they were forgiven. Laurisa read a poem she had written for her father. In turn, the grandson's mother gave Gavin Coffee's widow a bouquet of roses and they both sobbed. The grandfather told the Coffees he prayed every night for the children who lost their father. "It hurts like the devil," he said, crying. He blamed himself for not securing the load. His grandson also admitted he should have secured the load because he was the one driving.

In lieu of jail time, the men were sentenced to 200 hours of community service, specifically to educate others about "Maria's Law." They would report directly to Robin for one hundred hours and to Polly Young at King County Solid Waste for the other one hundred. They also were fined and would need to pay restitution.

When the media reported on the sentencing, it struck Heidi that her act of forgiving the two men was what made the story newsworthy, rather than the need to secure loads. How pathetic, Heidi thought, that forgiveness is so uncommon that it would be newsworthy. But if the accompanying story of Gavin's death made more people aware of unsecured loads, then she figured it was worthwhile.

When the papers discussed her husband's accident and the subsequent application of "Maria's Law" there were always readers who left anonymous on-line comments to the effect that

Gavin shouldn't have swerved. In a rare moment of bitterness, Heidi thought, Yeah, not swerving really worked out for Maria Federici.

Heidi keeps a photograph of Gavin on the mantle in the living room, watching over their children as they grow up without him. Heidi's youngest son Silas never met his father; her oldest daughter had been looking forward to having her dad teach her to drive. She knows that the two men who caused the accident are terribly sorry, perhaps even haunted by what happened. But the fact will always remains that because of their negligence she lost her husband, her children lost their father, and their future as a family was shattered. What could possibly constitute restitution for the loss of someone so beloved in the community, such a devoted father? Restitution might cover the value of the car, the deductible on the insurance, but not a man's life. Why, Heidi still asks herself, why don't people do the right thing without the threat of a fine to make them act differently?

The grandfather and grandson applied themselves diligently to their community service hours, always reporting to Robin and Polly Young exactly on time and doing whatever was asked of them. Young had them go to transfer stations to distribute "Secure Your Load" brochures and a write-up of the consequences of their failure to secure their load. The only time that Robin heard the grandson get angry was when he asked, "Why don't they teach all drivers to secure their load? Why isn't it part of Driver's Education?"

Robin had been working on that very issue. First, "Secure Your Load" had to become part of the Department of Licensing guidebook, and then it would become part of Driver's Education classes. The process of adding the law to the booklet took longer than Robin would have liked, but she finally accomplished it. Get it in writing first, she always figured, then it will have to be taught.

After sponsoring Maria's Law in the House of Representatives, Ruth Kagi thought it was tragically ironic that its first application, after Gavin Coffee's death, had to occur in her district. Then on October 4, 2005 the law became even more personal.

The Qamar and Kagi families had been close for years. Tony Qamar, the father, was traveling by car to the Olympic Peninsula, along with a colleague, to do seismic readings. Tony was the Washington State Seismologist, and a professor at the University of Washington. In front of them on the highway was a logging truck that, without warning, suddenly lost its full load of timber, completely crushing the Qamars' car. Tony and his colleague, Dan Johnson, died at the scene.

After the accident, Kagi learned there were no intrastate safety protocols for commercial trucks, so she sponsored legislation that would create them and allow the State Patrol to check for compliance. Drivers and companies would lose their commercial driving privileges if they didn't meet safety criteria. Tony's wife testified in Olympia, showing video footage of her husband's accident and of Tony at work. Tony's widow had become another safety advocate in the aftermath of the tragedy and Kagi was even more motivated to make roads less dangerous.

Spared lives rarely make headlines. There's no list of injuries and deaths prevented by Maria's Law. But when Kagi sees freeway signs reminding drivers to secure their loads, she is struck by what can be accomplished by people who transform personal tragedy into passion. Once, she even heard her daughter brag to a friend about "Secure Your Load" reminders.

"That's my mom's law," she said.

It's for Maria, it's for Gavin and for Tony and the families they left behind. It's a mom's law.

PART THREE

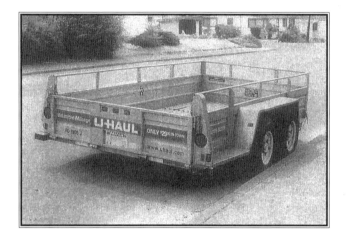

"It all began and ended with the RO Open Trailer..."
Simon H. Forgette, Esquire
Photo admitted as evidence Cause No. 06-02-11563

Starting with the Washington State Patrol's media blitz immediately after Maria was injured, both Robin and her daughter had benefited from sympathetic coverage and ongoing public interest. That changed somewhat when people heard they were filing a lawsuit against U-Haul. Written comments on articles posted on-line accused them of going after the company simply because it had "deep pockets." The suit, filed on April 4, 2006, included allegation of product liability against U-Haul and negligence against its registered agent Capron Holdings and the driver, James Hefley.

Robin tried not to care what people were saying about her and Maria. What would they do if their daughter were going to need lifelong medical care? Would they ignore the fact that a young man without insurance, using a suspended driver's license, had been allowed to rent a poorly designed open trailer and was sent on his way without special instructions about how to secure a load? Why did this suddenly make their campaign for safer roads through "Maria's Law" seem suspect overnight? Maria's incident had opened Robin's eyes to the dangers of unsecured loads and road debris; why should that message be compromised? What about all the other accidents in Washington every year because of road debris? What about the families of Sandy Harmon or Gavin Coffee?

A tort simply means a wrongful act. There was no question in Robin's mind that the circumstances of her daughter's injuries derived from a series of wrongful acts. Robin trusted that the facts would prevail, that the legal team could meet the burden of proof and show that Maria wouldn't have been injured on that roadway if the open trailer had been properly designed. What if the load couldn't be secured in the trailer despite the driver's best efforts?

Supporting Maria had always brought out the best in people, made heroes of ordinary citizens. Robin resolved to ignore criticism and focus on the heroes. For two years they had been living on Robin's savings. Her little house was almost paid for and she had always been frugal. Plus, she'd found so many treasures over the years at garage sales that she was still selling a few of her things. Heirloom quilts, sets of dishes. Every bit helped. The attorneys had warned her that even if they should prevail against U-Haul, it could be years before the company settled. Money remained from various benefits for Maria, but Robin was trying to make it last for several more years. The trial date was set for eighteen months in the future, September 17, 2007, which seemed too far away. The attorneys told Robin the trial date was a moving target, but she was adamant. "The trial date cannot change," she said. It became another mantra.

Simon Forgette gave numerous national presentations on the challenges of representing clients with brain injury. He had started his career as a JAG trial lawyer in the United States Marine Corps. When Robin told him about her daughter, Forgette realized that Maria would be the most severely injured person he had ever represented who was not either comatose or paraplegic. In the face of a mother's passion, he listened intently. But no matter how sympathetic he felt, he had to determine whether a case could be made for negligence or product liability. Unlike Robin, Forgette had a choice whether to get involved. His first step was to consult with his trusted longtime colleague, J. Murray Kleist.

Kleist had been threatening to retire for a dozen years, but there always seemed to be another big case on the horizon. The Federici case turned out to be his last before he really did let his license expire, but if it hadn't been for Kleist there might not have been a trial at all.

Kleist had been a personal injury attorney for fifty years. In his mind, an attorney representing an injured plaintiff is an entirely different breed than a defense attorney. A plaintiff's attorney doesn't get paid unless he wins the case. The defense attorney, on the other hand, is generally paid by the hour: win, lose or draw.

Forgette and Kleist had different styles. Kleist considered Forgette stately, whereas he viewed his own approach as decidedly flamboyant. But their philosophies were similar. Both men represented only plaintiffs—if they won their case, they got their contingency fee. They had to be good to keep working, and often the payoffs were far better than good. Forgette usually paid Kleist more than Kleist himself thought he had been worth to the case. "Whatever you think is fair," he'd tell Forgette.

When Forgette called Kleist about the Federici case, Kleist got excited. He had been in the business long enough to have heard about the questionable safety practices at U-Haul. As an airplane pilot he was familiar with aerodynamics, and the physics of the accident interested him. Forgette tended to be quite diligent about research before agreeing to act as counsel. Kleist offered to conduct his own investigation. Even before Forgette took the case, Kleist thought that to deal with such a big corporation they should team with defense attorney Bill Leedom—even though he was usually on "the other side."

The law offices of Forgette and his associate attorney, Janis Nevler, are tucked into a small office building in Kirkland, across from a waterfront park on Lake Washington. The offices are filled with antiques and paintings. All of Forgette's assistants work within hearing range and have been with him an average of twenty years. Forgette tries the cases in court; Nevler prefers to work behind the scenes.

Provided it has merit Forgette can afford to take on a case that may not be settled for years and cost tens of thousands of potentially unrecoverable dollars, but he has to help clients realize that they may have to survive for many years before a settlement is reached. That is why many cases with merit aren't tried; the client cannot survive that long and so accepts a settlement that may be far less than a jury would award.

The Federici case would be complicated and expensive. It would be a civil case, not criminal. Civil suits are based on tort law that helps to establish what can be reasonably expected from a product or a person's action. In a civil suit, a defendant may not have broken a law but they may have acted negligently or manufactured an unsafe product.

Some people believe that Americans are overly eager to sue, to blame a company for death or injury. But the less visible side of tort law is that lawsuits are often what forces a manufacturer to improve the safety of its products. They're what compel companies to build power tools with an automatic shut-off device, child seats with warnings about correct usage, windshields that don't shatter, or exit doors in buildings that stay illuminated when the power is out.

If a plaintiff is able to meet the "burden of proof" so that a jury finds that negligence occurred or that a product is unsafe, then the plaintiff will be able to collect compensatory damages. If the plaintiff is compensated, only then is the attorney also compensated – based on a percentage of the award. As Kleist likes to say, "We get paid if you get paid."

The contingency fee is sometimes referred to as the poor man's key to the court house. In Forgette's view the contingency fee system allows people without money a chance to have access to decent attorneys. Personal injury lawyers are sometimes characterized as ambulance chasers who encourage lawsuits. Forgette bristles at this.

"Attorneys will not generally take a case on contingency," he said, "unless they believe they can meet the burden of proof. This actually reduces frivolous law suits."

Forgette sized up the pros and cons of the Federici case. The damages potential was obviously huge; Maria's injuries were devastating and would be lifelong. Also there had been a police investigation with documented evidence of what had occurred. That was a plus. However U-Haul was self-insured and would be a difficult adversary.

Kleist looked over the notes with Forgette and suggested they look at the actual RO Open Trailer that was involved in the accident. Considering the driver's repeated insistence that he'd tied down the furniture that had escaped the trailer, could they prove product liability? Was the trailer obviously defective? The Washington State Patrol investigation file included the serial number of the trailer in question. Kleist and Carol Hodovance, one of Forgette's paralegals, drove to a Texaco Station in Bellevue owned by William Capron and rented the same RO trailer linked to Maria's accident.

When Kleist rented the trailer, no one gave him instructions on loading it, or asked what objects he planned to move. All the open trailers are what U-Haul calls "utility" trailers. The RO Open Trailer was simply the internal model name given to the six-foot by twelve-foot utility trailer first manufactured in 1999. Kleist picked up a safety brochure on his own. He hitched the trailer to his truck and drove to a spot just up the street from Forgette's office. Forgette then came out to examine it. He found it hard to believe that Kleist had so effortlessly rented the actual trailer involved in the accident.

Forgette figured he himself fit the profile of a typical U-Haul trailer renter, perhaps to take a daughter to college or to move a son into his first apartment. Like most people, he wouldn't have had a clue about appropriate knots to use or how to tie down a load. He noted that the trailer was huge, six-feet wide by twelve-feet long. But the side gates were only twenty-four-inches high. As for the back gate, it was only seventeen-inches high. Remarkably, there were no internal or floor tie-down points, no ropes provided, no nets, no loops through which to secure objects, just the side rails that were higher than the tail gate. His pulse quickened. As of that moment the case was no longer hypothetical. This trailer really wasn't safe, Forgette thought. We have a case.

Forgette and Kleist then turned to other questions. What if the driver had lost the load despite his best efforts? Had there been other accidents with these trailers? In investigating these and many related questions, the attorneys began to realize that if they could figure out the circumstances of the accident and prove product liability, they wouldn't be doing it just for Maria, but for thousands of people on the roadways.

CHAPTER

29

It took twenty months from the time Forgette agreed to represent Maria until the team, which included Bill Leedom, filed the complaint at King County Courthouse–almost two years of research before the real start of litigation. Their efforts bore no resemblance to a "frivolous lawsuit."

The complaint, filed in April, 2006, drew the battle lines. In order to defend its assets, U-Haul was going to need to pin part of the blame on Maria Federici and on its co-defendant James Hefley. The team realized that the driver needed to be U-Haul's fall guy.

If the jury found any or all of the defendants guilty of negligence and/or product liability, it would have to apportion each defendant a percentage of fault. To further complicate matters, Washington State honors what's called "joint and several liability." This meant that each party, no matter what their percentage of liability, was responsible for all of the damages. If one or more party could not pay, then the party that could was responsible for all damages. There was one huge caveat to this process: the injured party must be completely fault-free. In this case, if Maria was found to be so much as one percent responsible for her injuries, then "joint and several liability" would disappear. That would mean that each negligent party would be responsible for just its portion of the damages.

Although Hefley was one of the co-defendants, he would probably not have to pay all damages allocated to him; he declared bankruptcy before the trial started.

Lawsuits like Maria's can expose the plaintiff and their family to counter-accusations because the defense often tries to transform the "victim" into a "guilty party." Maria hated being labeled a victim almost as much as she hated being categorized as a blind person. As a plaintiff in the suit, she would become a target; it was the defense's job to prove she bore some responsibility for the accident, even though she was just driving home after work. Although Robin's family was still extremely supportive of her and Maria, Robin made a conscious decision to protect her family from the scrutiny that would come with the trial. She knew it was possible they might feel she was pushing them away but Robin preferred to protect them from photographers lurking in the bushes. She could only try to protect Maria during the trial, but her family she could at least spare.

"Try not to take these things personally," Jan Nevler counseled Robin. Over the years she would seem like a therapist to Robin.

"We've been through this before," Jan told her. "You haven't."

Robin could relax somewhat about the lawsuit, knowing she had hired experts in personal injury law. In between working with Norm's office on legislation and managing Maria's care, Robin worked on the endless checklist of items needed by Forgette's office, as lawyers began the investigation needed to prepare a complaint.

The complaint names a defendant or defendants, outlines the basics of the case, including its legal basis, identifies the injuries and specifies damages requested. The complaint is formally served to the defendant and filed with the court. The defendant then knows he's being sued, and why.

Cause No. 06-2-11-11563-5 SEA listed twenty-one Causes of Action against defendants U-Haul International, U-Haul Washington, Capron Holdings (the rental agent), and one against Hefley for negligence. The complaint in its entirety specified that the plaintiff intended to pursue damages and special damages, for medical costs to date and in the future, and loss of potential future earnings. The complaint was served on U-Haul along with a summons to trial, just as jurors for the case would later receive their special summons. Each defendant can then deny a certain allegation or even blame someone else.

The time between the complaint and the trial also includes "discovery," which is the preparation both sides do before trial, gathering information and evidence. Discovery can involve thousands of pieces of paper–engineering drawings, memos, white papers–just about anything either side thinks will be useful. Sometimes it involves searching for a needle in not just one haystack, but an entire field of haystacks. For their part, U-Haul wanted a detailed account of every time Robin had talked to a safety organization and a record of every bit of media coverage. Robin had warned Simon she wouldn't discontinue public speaking; and he knew better than to ask it of her. She might attempt to shield her family but campaign for public safety was simply too important.

Personal injury firms are generally small, like Forgette's, whereas defense attorney firms are usually bigger. Bennett, Bigelow & Leedom, for instance, a firm specializing in defense work, employs about twenty-five attorneys.

William Leedom was a partner in this firm and had extensive experience representing University of Washington physicians, which included those who worked at Harborview Medical Center. Leedom specialized in medical issues and had strong relationships with doctors. He also loved to do occasional plaintiff work. Unlike Simon, he didn't mind media attention, which would be another benefit to having him on board for the trial. Simon, Murray and Bill had all worked together on a major case—and been very successful. For all these reasons, Forgette and Kleist thought he would make an ideal co-counsel.

For someone known as feisty and extremely competitive, Bill Leedom doesn't look that imposing. He's built like an athlete, and has slightly faded sandy skin coloring. He ran regularly during the trial no matter the weather. Like almost everyone else involved in the case, he's from the Northwest. He has daughters about Maria's age and, best of all for Robin, is devoted to golden retrievers. Robin had signed a retainer agreement with his firm after Forgette explained why co-counsel would be needed. Combining plaintiff and defense attorneys on their team would give them extra insight and strength in taking on an international corporation.

Before he could accept the assignment, however, Leedom had to persuade his partners that the potential financial risks of the case would be justified. He would be taking staff away from billable defense work to toil for years on a contingency fee case. Although his argument must have been compelling, if Leedom had known what would come out during discovery, he might not have been able to talk his partners into accepting the case.

Jan Nevler lived and breathed the Federici case for years. Like so many others on the team, Nevler grew up in Seattle, got her law degree in Seattle, and has practiced locally for twenty-five years. She's also a parent; her older daughter just passed her driving test. As a personal injury specialist, Nevler knows how quickly life can change, and that she cannot keep her daughters safe at every moment. She has versed her husband

and daughters in the importance of securing loads, and predicts that her daughters will become proselytizers for the cause, as she has.

At family functions, around the barbeque in the summer, or at the Thanksgiving table, she would ask, "What would you think about an open trailer that doesn't have tie-downs?" Nevler's brother, George, and his friends were the type of people who would choose to move heavy objects in a do-it-yourself fashion, U-Haul's target audience. She'd grill them: "Would you rent an open trailer without tie-downs?" George became as vigilant about enforcing "Secure Your Load" as anyone. He worked for Washington State Ferries, and if he noticed trucks on the vehicle deck with unsecured loads, he would have them pull over to the side to "button it down," and instructed his crew to do the same. "He was one small foot soldier for the cause," Nevler said. For two years Nevler and all of her extended local family lived the Federici case, as the office prepared the suit, went through discovery, and made the long journey to the trial.

Nevler considered it her job to provide emotional support for the clients. In a law office focused on personal injury and product liability, the clients always have multiple needs, from immediate financial to long-term social and emotional.

"It's part of our role to remind them of what the outcome might be," she said. "Even if the case is over and we win, not everything is going to be all better. Their healing process is going to be ongoing."

Nevler's primary role in the Federici case was to go through U-Haul documents once they were wrested from corporate headquarters, and all of the medical records. During discovery she also had to track down items requested by U-Haul, such as a record of every single news item, interview, and speaking engagement as it related to Maria or Robin since the accident.

U-Haul's witness list was incredibly long, and Nevler was astonished by all the angles that the U-Haul defense seemed to be pursuing based on their requests. She tried to anticipate the most important themes in the trial, and what kind of evidence U-Haul would produce. She and Kleist went through every trailer design they could acquire. In their research of other cases and claims, they found references to many objects that had fallen from U-Haul trailers, from pianos to furniture and toolboxes.

In Nevler's work she thinks a lot about how people react to a tragedy, and has often witnessed people who use tragedy as a catalyst or springboard. "Certain people see the bigger picture," she said. "It's remarkable how ordinary people can elevate themselves into doing the extraordinary." The family of a child who died because his seat belt didn't restrain him during an accident went on to create legislation that makes booster seats mandatory. That family had been their clients.

Like Forgette, Nevler thinks often about the litany of safety features that resulted from lawsuits–product warning labels and the like. "Brought to you by that much vilified group," she mused, "trial lawyers." In her sensible way, Nevler said, without apparent judgment, "Industry doesn't always do the best job of regulating itself."

After Bill Leedom convinced his partners to take the Federici case, the bulk of the early preparation work went to legal assistant Cate Brewer and a first-year attorney named Tim Allen. Cate Brewer was almost a rarity in that she had not heard of Maria Federici before she started work on the case, simply because she and her family were still living in Montana in 2004. As for Tim Allen, he was not your average freshman attorney in a Seattle law firm. He had been Professor of Political Philosophy and Argumentation for sixteen years at

Western Washington University, in Bellingham, and Director of Western's debate team. He thought of the Federici trial preparation as particularly fun, with the exception of a week spent in Phoenix, Arizona, attempting to get records from U-Haul's corporate offices, with an average daily temperature over one hundred degrees.

As a person who welcomed a good debate, Allen thought that U-Haul was a worthy opponent. The company was prepared to fight every lawsuit thrown at it, big or small. When Allen visited U-Haul in Phoenix, company officials resisted providing documents he requested, which didn't seem to Allen like an intelligent strategy. Allen and a colleague were looking for information on the RO Trailer that Hefley used the night of Maria's accident–engineering documents, safety testing, and incident reports. After acquiring a subpoena from the King County Prosecutor's Office, U-Haul finally produced documents that showed hundreds of references to incidents involving U-Haul equipment, and others involving open trailers in the ten years before the first RO Trailer.

As both sides prepare for trial, each side can attempt to narrow the case by amending the complaint. This can lead to what is called motion practice, whereby one side seeks relief from the judge. If a motion asks for the court to make a finding based on a matter of law, that calls for a summary judgment. There are motions and counter-motions. Before Maria's trial concluded, Tim Allen had worked on ninety-five separate motions.

30

It was in May of 2007 that U-Haul and Nevler received records from Harborview Hospital that raised a lot of eyebrows and spun the trial preparation into a completely new direction. A blood panel conducted on Maria indicated above-average blood-alcohol content when she arrived at the hospital via Medic One immediately following her injury.

Maria's legal team suspected that U-Haul would wield the test results like a smoking gun. So Leedom began contacting medical experts about the validity of the test. U-Haul moved to amend their answer to the complaint to include in their defense that Maria was intoxicated at the time of the accident. U-Haul's action was front-page news. The Harborview test was a big challenge for Maria's team and a windfall for U-Haul. It gave the defense a reason to request an extension of the trial date, though Forgette and Leedom fought to keep the original date, as Robin insisted.

By the time Robin's deposition date drew near, she was working more and more closely with the legal team. They kept her apprised of what they learned during discovery, and met with her the week before she and Maria were scheduled to be deposed by U-Haul's counsel. As usual, Kleist's assessment of the goal of their deposition was blunt. "It's not that they don't know the answer to the question," he told Robin and Maria.

"They just need to get it on the record so you can't weasel out of it later."

The curse and blessing of Maria's brain injuries was that she tended to think that she was "fine." Anyone who had known her before the accident was at once amazed by how much she had recovered, but also by her lack of awareness at how greatly she had changed. In her deposition, Maria would likely paint a fairly rosy picture of her life, because she didn't have the capacity to see the extent of her disabilities.

Robin was always torn between protecting her daughter's self-image and addressing the realities of her situation. A magazine had wanted to run a headline that used Maria's beauty in the past tense. "My daughter is still beautiful," Robin protested, and the wording was changed. Robin couldn't pretend that Maria was fine. There was no one else as qualified to speak to the extent of Maria's disability. Just as children and adults with attention-deficit disorder are highly intelligent and compelled to mask their disabilities, Maria could appear more capable over short time periods than she could over the long haul. And Robin had been there for every day of the long haul.

Robin had been warned the defense attorneys would try to rattle and possibly attack her. Maria was the plaintiff but it was Robin's campaign to secure her daughter's financial survival. By now it had been over three years since the accident. How many more years could they survive?

The deposition was taken in the defense attorney's offices. As Robin waited in the impersonal lobby, she fingered a jade rock from her desk at home. She'd read in a book called "The Secret" that having an object to hold in stressful situations provides focus and power.

Maria had done her deposition a week earlier, without Robin. Forgette and Leedom had wanted Robin to be there with her, but Robin decided against it. Robin really wanted Maria to understand that her mother believed she could do it on her own. Maria wanted and needed to be more independent. Plus, Robin hadn't wanted the defense attorneys to have a chance to study her beforehand in case it gave them ideas on how to unsettle her during her own deposition. Robin was happy that Maria felt that her deposition had gone well.

The lead attorney for the defense was Patrick W. Schmidt from Quarles & Brady, a firm based in Milwaukee, Wisconsin. His local counterpart was Carl P. Gilmore of K&L Gates, with offices on the twenty-ninth floor of a downtown Seattle building. That's where the deposition took place. Years before, Robin had been deposed as a fact witness for a client at Wells Fargo, but it had never been personal before. Now she was fighting for her daughter's future.

Forgette and Nevler were also there, literally on her side of the table. On the other side were Schmidt and Gilmore for U-Haul, and a lawyer named Jim Howard, representing Capron Holdings. A court reporter was on hand to transcribe every word. Below the table, Robin stroked her lovely piece of jade, which she'd found at an antique sale.

The defense attorneys started with questions about her home and whether her parents were still living. Then they jumped to questions that seemed to reveal an area they planned to exploit at the trial–Robin's speaking engagements on the subject of "Secure Your Load."

Schmidt asked, "At any time, in any of your speeches or any of your public appearances, do you recall saying anything about the need for manufacturers of pickup trucks, or trailers, or cargo carriers, or other vehicles to change their design?"

"No," Robin replied.

"Why is that?"

"It's not my expertise." Robin said.

"Your expertise is in securing loads," Schmidt said, part statement, part question.

"My expertise is sharing our story," Robin said. Robin had always told audiences that she couldn't tell them how to secure a load, only to imagine people they loved driving in the car behind them.

He's trying to get me flustered, Robin reminded herself. I can't let him succeed. He wants me to take this personally. It's not personal for him—it's just business. Almost as though he read her thoughts, Schmidt, in the middle of asking Robin to admit she was upset with Hefley, said, "On a personal level, I am very sorry about what happened to your daughter."

"So am I," Robin said, "every day that I look at her."

Robin and the defense attorney both needed a break to regain their composure.

After the break Schmidt asked Robin about training for the blind that Robin had arranged for Maria. Robin was careful to take her time forming answers, remembering to breathe calmly. His questions made her feel defensive. "Has anyone told you that the dog she has is not the best kind of dog to be used as a therapy dog?" Schmidt asked. "Sammy is not a service dog, correct? Why has there not been an effort to contact those folks who do have, as I understand it, services available for non-sighted people?"

Based on the lawyer's questions, Robin thought she could identify what his themes would be in the trial. Let's show that the mother speaks frequently on the need for people to secure their loads, as though implying that the trailer was not at fault but rather the person who didn't secure the load. Let's show the mother isn't "allowing" Maria to be institutionalized for occupational training. Let's show that the mother could be working full-time, that her daughter's medical condition doesn't really warrant her full-time care.

Robin wished the questions would end. Schmidt asked, "If Mr. Hefley had borrowed a pickup truck and had used it to haul the entertainment center and it fell out, would you blame the pickup manufacturer?"

"I don't know," Robin said.

"Object to form," Forgette interjected, but Schmidt pressed on.

"Then why are you blaming U-Haul in this case?" he asked. "If you are. Maybe you're not. Maybe you don't believe U-Haul is at fault. You tell me."

Strangely, the more that Forgette voiced his objections to the forms of the questions, the calmer Robin felt. It seemed less personal to her that Schmidt tried to get her to say U-Haul's role was incidental, that it was the driver who had been completely at fault.

"What on earth does the fact that Mr. Hefley doesn't have insurance have to do with whether he did or didn't secure his load?" Schmidt asked.

Robin replied that she felt that U-Haul was partially responsible for the accident by renting the driver an open trailer without proper instructions or proper equipment, and hadn't checked to see whether he had a valid driver's license or insurance. This was negligent behavior in Robin's view.

Then Schmidt played the hand he'd been holding. "Did you read this morning's newspapers?" he asked.

Robin told him no.

"Are you aware that the papers have put on the front page, at least one of them, the contents of the lab report from Harborview Hospital?"

"No," Robin said. "I wasn't aware they had done that."

She tried to stay calm, even though she wanted to rage. Leedom had explained the blood-alcohol test to her and how U-Haul might publicize it even though it was probably a false-positive, triggered by massive blood loss and organ failure.

"I want you to assume for a moment, Ms. Abel," Schmidt said, "that in fact your daughter had a 0.124 blood alcohol content on the night of the accident. Would you attribute some blame to this accident to her?"

Robin could just imagine her reply being taken out of context. He was asking her to answer as though Maria was legally drunk? How could he ask her something like that?

"I don't believe she did." Robin said strongly.

"That's not my question."

"Object to the form," Forgette said again.

Schmidt circled the alcohol issue several times, asking about Maria's favorite drink, asking if Robin had ever gotten behind the wheel of a car when affected by alcohol, and asking whether it was true she'd likened the "Secure Your Load" campaign to the "Mothers Against Drunk Driving" campaign.

He was trying to connect her outreach on "Maria's Law" with the issue of drunk driving, as though the connection was drinking, not a mother's passionate mission because of what had happened to her child.

"You have the personal view," Schmidt pressed, "that people who have blood-alcohol content above the legal limit in the State of Washington should not be driving, correct?"

"I guess I would agree," Robin said. She hated that he was implying that if Maria's blood alcohol content was above the legal limit that Robin would believe she shouldn't have been on the road that night, and was somehow responsible for the accident. Forgette had warned her that U-Haul would try hard to show that Maria was even partially liable, because if Maria was liable for even one percent it would get them off the hook for some of the damages.

Then Schmidt switched gears again.

"Sitting here under oath today, Ms. Abel, will you agree with me that one of the real reasons that U-Haul is being sued in this case is because Mr. Hefley didn't have insurance and you see U-Haul as being a 'deep pocket'?"

"No!" Robin said.

Schmidt backed off again and worked his way through the witness list, clarifying relationships. Then suddenly he asked,

"What does your daughter do for fun?"

Robin's jaw dropped. It was so inappropriate. She wanted to scream: Fun, what fun? She's blind. She can't smell. She can't taste. She has severe brain damage. She has constant sick headaches. She can't open her mouth more than a quarter of an inch. What fun?

"Not much," Robin replied with a tinge of sarcasm. Not much was left of her daughter's life from before the accident, and he dared to ask what she did for "fun?"

Robin could see that Schmidt had tears welling up behind his thick glasses. He stood up and pushed back his chair. "Let's take a break," he said as he left the room.

Robin turned to Forgette, "Did you see his tears?"

Forgette had been taking notes and hadn't seen his face. But Robin had seen them.

The worst was over. After nearly three hours, Schmidt finally said, "I think that's all I have."

Robin was relieved the deposition was over, but the defense attorney had tipped her to the ugliness waiting outside of the conference room, spurred by the news story. When Robin picked up the Seattle Post-Intelligencer, she winced at the headline: "U-Haul Claims Federici Drunk at Time of Accident."

Much later, when Maria's blood-alcohol results were ruled completely invalid by the court, newspapers didn't print a story with the headline: "Federici Sober at Time of Accident." No, the defense had started their efforts to discredit the plaintiff months before the trial, and for some people that headline stuck forever. Maria's legal team had warned Robin that U-Haul would fight hard. How could she have been naïve enough to think that fighting hard meant fighting fair?

The day after Robin's deposition, it was as though the earth itself had opened and the bottom fell out of her world again.

CHAPTER
31

Norm Maleng planned to work until the day he died, and he did. He'd said that he wanted to be buried in his business suit, and he was. As per his wishes, he was buried in the family plot in his hometown of Acme, next to Karen.

Norm went to Mariners' spring training every year but otherwise he loved his work too much to take many vacations. During the holidays, when most of his staff was out of the office, he loved to go in to catch up on paperwork and prepare for the new calendar year. Norm was always prepared. But the Malengs had always wanted to go to Norway. For Judy's sixtieth birthday they were really going to make the trip. Even though it was a beautiful night on May 24th they felt obligated to attend a fundraising dinner for the Scandinavian Department at the University of Washington. As the highest ranking government official who would be in attendance, Norm had been asked to deliver the toast for a visiting Norwegian ambassador.

At the Urban Horticulture Center they strolled the outside courtyard waiting until it was time to go inside for dinner. Suddenly Norm said to Judy, "I need to sit down. I feel dizzy." Judy looked for a seat but benches were a few feet away.

"I've got you," she said, holding onto him.

He started to collapse and some men entering the courtyard saw she needed help. Together they helped to lay him out on the ground. One man said, "Should I call 9-1-1?" Another man that Judy recognized lifted Norm's wrist to feel for a pulse, looking at his watch in a professional manner, like a nurse or doctor. Judy made the mistake of thinking that he knew exactly what he was doing; that moment still haunts her. She thought Norm was breathing; she learned later that it may have been a reflex in the epiglottis. The man who called 9-1-1 said "a gentleman had fainted." Is that why it took so long before she heard the sirens? With Norm on the ground, eyes closed, those minutes were the longest of her life. She ran out to the fire truck where a firefighter seemed to be taking his time pulling out his gear.

"Hurry," she yelled. "Please hurry."

"Dispatch said someone had fainted," he said.

"No! It's much more," Judy said.

The medics worked on him in the garden long enough for their son to drive across town to be with them. When the Medic One truck pulled out, Norm was raced to Harborview instead of University Hospital, which was closer. The paramedics, recognizing that Norm was going to need the most intensive response available, knew that only Harborview could provide it. After all, Harborview and Medic One had put Seattle on the map as the safest place in the nation to have a heart attack, making the difference between life and death for Maria.

Word that Norm was on his way to Harborview preceded his arrival there. It turned out that another guest at the fundraiser, a King County judge, had telephoned Dan Satterberg, and he in turn had called the other King County division heads, along with Susan Gregg-Hanson, the head of Harboview's media relations department. By the time Medic One got to Harborview, Satterberg was already there, along with King County Executive Ron Sims, Seattle Chief of Police Gil Kerlikowske, and Norm's top deputies.

Dr. Copass was also on hand, because there were standing orders at Harborview to call him if someone of Norm's stature were on his way into emergency.

"We're going to save Norm," Copass told the director of Harborview as they waited for the Medic One vehicle.

Judy and Mark watched as Copass gave commands to his medical department staff.

"You will do what I tell you to do when I tell you to do it," Copass ordered.

A man was on her husband's chest giving him compressions. It's been too long, Judy thought. Norm is not going to live. It had been hours since he first told her that he needed to sit down.

The time of death was noted as 9:11 p.m.

The morning after Maleng's death, the entire prosecuting attorney's office gathered in the ninth-floor courtroom. "Norm would want us to carry on," the division chiefs told the five hundred attorneys and staffers. From building security guards on up, everyone simply loved Norm. He would chat with the guards about the Mariners season and he knew about their families. Each day one of Norm's assistants would ensure that he made time for his ritual lunch, a tuna salad sandwich and a carton of milk. Norm was often the first to arrive in the morning, but never the last to leave. Unless he had a meeting, he was always home for dinner. On Norm's desk there were notes from his final meeting–with the Eastside Domestic Violence Unit. On a lined yellow pad on his desk at home were notes for a vestry meeting at his church. He was always prepared. "Let me think about it over the weekend and get back to you on Monday," Norm would tell his staff when they proposed a new idea.

Norm's division heads had a succession plan worked out by the following Monday. Dan Satterberg, Norm's Chief of Staff for seventeen years, would serve as Interim Prosecuting

Attorney, until the King County Council could confirm him as Acting Prosecuting Attorney. He would plan to run in the next election.

Robin was one of thousands who mourned Maleng across the state. In June she attended his memorial service, where she noticed that his date of birth, September 17, was the same date that Maria's trial was scheduled to start. She felt more strongly than ever that the trial date must not be moved. If the trial began on his birthday, it would mean that Norm was still watching over her.

During the summer following Norm's death, Judy Maleng got a message on her answering machine from someone she didn't recognize. The message said, "Judy, I'm sorry for calling you, but Norm was always there for me. I'm Maria Federici's mom."

Judy remembered that Norm had once come home from work with a box in his hand. He had told her that Robin and Maria had been to visit and asked him to give her the box. Inside was a beautiful beaded bracelet Maria had made. Judy wondered at the time, how could someone blind create something so intricate?

Judy knew that Robin and Maria had been very important to Norm; he'd felt a connection to Maria. When Judy called Robin back, they spoke for an hour, both of them emotional, trading stories about Norm and how much they missed him—and their daughters. Robin invited her to the cabin. Judy made the hour-long drive on a lovely sunny day. She stopped on the way and picked up sandwiches. When she arrived, Robin bounced out to meet her as the dogs barked.

"Welcome," Robin said, tears in her eyes.

They took chairs and sat on the dock. Lake Kathleen and Robin's property seemed so distant from Seattle. "This is the life," Judy said. Being with Robin and Maria, meeting them both for the first time, reminded Judy of what she knew in her heart, that life goes on after tragedy, the perennials return, the zinnias and snapdragons thrive, butterflies swoop, and the sun's warmth can still feel like a gift.

At the end of her visit, Judy told Robin, "I can't be Norm but I will try and be there for you the way he would have been."

Far away from the lake and garden, the battle over the blood-alcohol test dominated the legal proceedings leading up to the September trial. Bill Leedom asked Dr. Copass to prepare a declaration on the matter for the Federici case. It was to be submitted at a hearing on its admissibility as evidence. Copass agreed, and based on a review of relevant medical journals and Maria's file, he concluded that the tests results were not reliable. On July 17, Copass was questioned under oath about his declaration, by Lisa Marchese, an attorney for U-Haul and Capron Holdings, as part of the pre-trial motions.

Physicians, like other professionals, tend to use acronyms freely. Some are shorthand for trauma tests; others refer to chemicals by their molecular breakdown, such as ETOH for ethanol. AOB is short for Alcohol-On-Breath and BAL for Blood-Alcohol Level. Copass explained that blood-serum panels are run on most patients who arrive due to severe trauma or with AOB. Maria's trauma panel was a standard test; it was not administered because of any indication of alcohol on her breath. The results are displayed in a graph that assigns different colors to different chemicals. The enzyme machine assigns the same color coding to alcohol as to the enzyme called NADH Dehydrogenase. NADH Dehydrogenase is commonly produced when a patient has severe blood loss. At first glance, it might appear that Maria had an elevated blood-alcohol level because of the lack of differentiation in color coding. She had definitely had severe blood loss.

The test that appeared to indicate the presence of alcohol, Copass explained, was just part of standard testing on trauma patients, and used blood serum, not whole blood. It was not ordered for "forensic" or criminal purposes, but just for establishing a data point to determine how to best treat the patient.

His testimony and that of Dr. Chandler, Chief of Service for Laboratory Medicine at Harborview, was very technical. When a patient's blood loss is severe, their organs and tissues are deprived of oxygen; this is known as ischemia. During ischemia, chemical changes occur in a person's blood serum, altering albumin and causing concentrations to rise quickly and remain elevated for several hours. This is what caused the elevated NADH Dehydrogenase.

Copass referred to the fact Maria was in "catastrophic metabolic condition" at the time of the blood draw. An enzyme test that assigns various colors to chemicals in the blood could not be deemed reliable at such a stage. The manufacture of the testing machine had even noted in its literature that NADH could be falsely read as alcohol. Copass restated his written conclusion that the test results for certain blood factors were unreliable and unscientific for all purposes.

He cited scientific literature documenting that high lactate levels interfere with enzymatic testing, such as the one to detect ETOH. For perspective, Copass said that Maria had the highest level of lactate seen in the ER in many, many years. "Her lactic of 13.5 may be the highest I've ever seen in a person who survived, other than a septic individual," he said. "In an individual so severely injured, that may be the highest I've ever seen."

Despite the countering arguments from Copass, if Maria's legal team had known beforehand that the Harborview blood-gas test would open the door to U-Haul accusing Maria of having elevated blood alcohol, the lawyers might not have taken on the case. The cost of counteracting the misleading test results might have been deemed too high, even in the face of strong evidence for product liability. Now there was a possibility that the defense could prove that plaintiff might have been even slightly responsible for the accident which affected all the formulas for joint and several liability. By the time the blood-alcohol test was discovered, Maria's legal team was too far down the road to turn back. It certainly raised the stakes, and made the team more focused than ever on scrupulous preparation.

On August 16, King County Superior Court Judge Glenna Hall granted the plaintiff's motion not to allow the blood serum-alcohol test from Harborview to be part of trial evidence. Her ruling was a big win for Maria's team. However the defense was allowed to introduce evidence about the glass of wine she consumed at the end of her shift with her supervisor Mason even though in his deposition he had testified that she showed no signs of impairment. By coincidence he had even followed her vehicle for several miles until his exit.

Bill Leedom issued a statement to the media: "The judge's decision is important to Maria because we can now focus on the real issues of the case: Was the open trailer defectively designed and did U-Haul fail to warn of the consequences of not securing a load properly?"

The Seattle Times didn't even report on the judge's ruling, letting stand their previous story that suggested the possibility Maria had been intoxicated. At least the Seattle Post-Intelligencer's story on the ruling softened the blow to Maria's character made by its initial story on the test. The headline read "Federici's Alcohol Level Can't Be Used."

After nearly two years of preparation, the trial was now imminent. Maria's legal team felt ready, especially after enduring so many pre-trial motions. Although each of the attorneys had a different way of describing the team's strategy, the gist was to put U-Haul's safety practices on trial. For the company's sixtieth anniversary in 2005, the public relations department had created a special logo that put the name U-Haul above the words "finest" and "safest."

"If U-Haul is going to take the position that safety is their trademark," Leedom explained, "then they need to show how they do that. If they don't rent properly designed equipment and provide safety instructions, they're creating danger for the general public. So how is safety their number-one priority?"

CHAPTER

32

The Federici trial was to be King County Superior Court Judge Glenna Hall's last major trial before retiring. She had been on the bench since 1987, serving first as Judge and Commissioner Pro Tempore through 1996, and then exclusively as Judge. Her interests outside the courtroom included singing, flying planes, and birdwatching. She reminded at least one of the jurors of his grandmother.

On September 17, 2007, what would have been Norm Maleng's sixty-ninth birthday, the trial started with the task of selecting a jury from a pool of nearly three hundred citizens. Against incredible odds, the initial trial date had not changed.

One of the defense attorneys, Lisa Marchese, was quoted in The Seattle Times regarding another case, "You can lose a case in jury selection. One mistake, one wrong choice, and it can affect the entire outcome." Within days, Maria's future care would be in the hands of the chosen jurors. Among them were a librarian, an attorney, a scientist, a park department worker, and two Microsoft employees. These twelve jurors, plus four alternates, would start the trial as strangers and end it as intimate acquaintances. They were told the trial was expected to last seven weeks–an eternity compared to the two-to-seven days that most jurors serve.

Robin felt like she had been waiting for her time in court ever since it became apparent that Maria was going to survive.

For twenty-four years her role as a mother had defined her life. Since the accident, Robin had been trying to fix her daughter, bone by bone, memory by memory, simultaneously surviving each day and trying to figure out how to secure the rest of her daughter's days. It was natural to want to be able to blame one person; not that it did any good. It was fact–what had happened to Maria could have been prevented. People who didn't know the facts claimed the lawsuit was about "deep pockets." For Robin it was about safety. Every load needed to have a means of being secured, whether it was hauled by rental trailers or trucks. In her opinion U-Haul shouldn't be allowed to put products in the hands of just anyone, without checking for a valid driver's license or proof of insurance. The company claimed that safety was its number one concern, but Robin didn't buy it. The evidence made Robin doubt that U-Haul cared who was driving one of its rentals, or who might be in the vehicles behind.

At last, everything that had transpired since that awful night three years before would be revealed in court, along with testimony about U-Haul's safety record. The defense planned to put Robin herself on trial, as a caregiver and safety advocate. Robin was ready; in fact she was as determined as she had ever been in her life.

Robin wasn't in the courtroom during jury selection, but the timing was perfect. She would have missed the trial for only one reason in the world and this happened to be it: the Governor's Annual Safety Conference which coincided with the start of the trial. After first attending the conference as one little mother in an almost empty booth, she was returning for her third year, this time as one of the main speakers.

As she was driving to the conference her car was hit by a two-by-four, which fortunately didn't break the windshield. Someone else might have thought it was an incredible coincidence, but Robin felt like obstacles were thrown at her every single day. This one was just a little more obvious. She saw debris every day on the roadways, as well as unsecured loads. She would approach drivers if she noticed a vehicle with a dangerous load in a parking lot. She had even gotten her first speeding ticket for passing an old jalopy with an unsecured load on an exit ramp that made her nervous. After the officer wrote the ticket she said to him, "I'd like you to do something for me. Talk to the rest of your officers about unsecured loads." When he asked her why, she replied, "I'm Maria Federici's mother." He looked stricken and encouraged her to go to court to get the fine reduced. "I deserved the ticket," she said. "But the other driver was the one who was dangerous." Robin had to believe that everyone who heard her message about unsecured loads would look at their own habits differently. They would secure their own load, or at least move away from a vehicle that looked dangerous on the roadway. How many people needed to be injured or killed before people changed their behavior? Robin would love to be able to just drive or even walk on a single day without noticing something dangerous–the neighbors loading firewood, the city truck with loose trash cans in the back. Just one single day! Would it be too much to ask?

Both sides made opening statements on Friday, September 21, outlining what they intended to present over the course of testimony. Bill Leedom displayed a map of the United States and used push pins to show where there had been similar incidents involving U-Haul's RO open trailer. Plaintiffs would emphasize liability and negligence, on the part of U-Haul and its agents, in the design of the open trailer and lack of warnings.

Pat Schmidt opened for U-Haul. "We won't dispute the tragedy here or the severity of the initial injuries but there is rebuilding that can be done," he said. His team would show evidence that Maria was following too closely to the vehicle in front of her and wouldn't have been as injured if she had ducked. He concluded, "The bottom line is what lies ahead for Federici is not the life of dependency on others, as plaintiffs suggest, but a plan for self-sufficiency if she gets the help she needs."

Lisa Marchese made opening statements for Capron Holdings, U-Haul's authorized agents at the Bellevue gas station that had rented the trailer to Hefley. "Ladies and gentlemen," she said, addressing the jury. "I submit to you that the evidence is going to show one thing. Capron Holdings had nothing to do with these horrible events that we all recognize."

James Hefley was unrepresented and appeared only for his testimony as an adverse witness. Maria's team of three attorneys—Leedom, Forgette and Allen—sat with Robin at the front table, facing the judge. The defense attorneys were to their left, and the jury box was to their right. Throughout the case, the spectator seats in this courtroom, King County's largest, were always filled. Plaintiffs presented their case first.

Robin watched the jurors' faces. If they had been ignorant of the case beforehand, they got a brutal introduction on the first day of testimony–a Friday. Jean Gamboa, the woman who'd stopped behind Maria on I-405, was the first witness. If her testimony was disturbing, then Dr. Westhoff's was horrifying. He described how blood was everywhere in the emergency department from Maria's injuries and how he began calling desperately for help. He told about the life-and-death surgery on her brain performed right in the emergency room. He had served in Iraq, yet said he'd never seen anything worse until that night in Harborview.

Westhoff was followed on the witness stand by Anthony Cox, the Metro driver who had broken into Maria's car and held her hand until the aid trucks arrived. Robin wished she could have spared him from recounting the events of that night. Cox described his habit of staying alert while driving by observing the actions of other drivers around him. He recalled pacing Maria's black Liberty to his right, and described how he saw its brake lights go on and sparks issue from it. He then slowed as her Jeep did, and pulled ahead to park some sixty feet in front of her car. When he spoke about what he saw inside the car, Cox became upset and couldn't continue for several minutes.

Then he explained the diagram he had drawn, the day after the accident, to show State Patrol investigators the sequence of events. His statement to the Patrol was referenced: "My clothes were covered with shards of glass and some blood. I threw away the clothes I was wearing. That night I could not sleep. My adrenalin was running high and my mind could not come to completion. I wanted to know how the victim was doing. I kept praying for her health. I just wanted to know if I made a difference."

His ongoing anguish was palpable. Robin wished she could say to Anthony then and there, "You made all the difference." She felt terrible that Cox was still so traumatized. Now the jurors had to think about what he had witnessed. As the judge sent them home for the weekend, she reminded the jurors not to speak about what they had heard to anyone, not even to each other.

Each day the court was in session, Robin would set her alarm for 4:00 a.m. so that she could curl her hair and put on her banker's outfit. Maria's caregiver would arrive later in the day for their regular routines of walking and going to the gym. Maria was at the stage where she could be alone for a few hours, but Robin always worried about her using the stove. Robin would be on the road to Kirkland by no later than 6:15, earlier if bad weather might slow down traffic. There she would meet Forgette, Kleist, and Forgette's assistant, Patty Pease, to carpool to the courthouse. If Forgette was in the courtroom, then Patty was there too. They usually left for Seattle at 8:00 a.m., in Forgette's older Mercedes. As a dog person, Robin came to see Maria's legal team as three breeds of canine. Forgette was the English mastiff, Kleist was the bulldog, and Leedom was the golden retriever. She loved them all. During the morning rides, they talked about the case. Sitting together in the courtroom, they couldn't nudge each other or speak openly; it wasn't until the commute back to Kirkland that they could speak freely again.

The day that William Capron testified, they couldn't talk about anything else. Even though he'd been a commissioned U-Haul agent through his gas station for twenty years, and had gotten one of the first RO Trailers produced, he said he'd never received specific information from U-Haul on how to secure trailer loads or the consequences of not doing so.

"To be honest," he testified, "I never actually thought about somebody following a trailer I had rented. . . ." Capron denied ever hearing about any of the incidents that Leedom had marked with push pins on the map during his opening statement, which marked the scenes of eight accidents involving open trailers before Maria's, and three since. Explaining why he and his employees didn't provide directions on securing open trailer loads, Capron said, under oath, "I think you'd be hard-pressed to find anybody in this building that wouldn't know how to load an open trailer. You know, I might be proven wrong on that, but I think everybody knows that if you don't tie it down, anything can come out."

Later, back in the Mercedes for the drive back to Kirkland, Kleist asked, "Did you see the looks on the faces of the women in the jury?"

"Not just the women!" Patty responded.

Capron had almost unwittingly addressed a key issue in the trial. Since there was a law that made it a crime if an unsecured load injured someone, didn't a company that targeted "do-it-yourself" movers have a responsibility to make sure loads could actually be secured—whether by design, extra equipment, or instruction?

"I guess everybody's supposed to understand aerodynamics and tensile strength," Kleist said to the group. ("Tensile strength" indicates the ability of rope to resist breaking.)

Those daily commutes in the Mercedes were Robin's favorite part of the day. For the first time in nearly four years, at least since Maria had left Harborview, she felt like part of a team. Although it felt cold enough to see your breath in Forgette's car after the heater broke, it was the warmest Robin had felt inside for years. After they parted outside of the Kirkland office, Robin would get into her Volkswagen Beetle and head for home in the peak of traffic. That's when she would always call her parents to tell them about the day in court. By the time Robin got home she was ready to take a break from the trial, but she always told Maria something about the day. Maria showed interest, but no more than if Robin had been attending the trial of a stranger and was just recounting her day. Then the next day the alarm would ring at 4:00 a.m. and she would do it all over again.

Robin felt it was her duty to be present at the trial every day, with two exceptions. She stayed at home when James Hefley spent an entire day on the stand, and she stepped out of the courtroom during Dr. Hopper's testimony. Everyone in the courtroom was forewarned that Hopper's presentation would be graphic in the worst sense of the word. Robin had vowed never to look at the photos of her faceless daughter. She knew that, once viewed, the images could never be unviewed. Hopper proved to be an extremely attractive and disarming witness despite his content, though the judge had to admonish him not to address the jury directly, after Hopper warned them that many of his PowerPoint slides would be gruesome.

When one of the jurors flatly stated that she wouldn't look at the slides, Hopper, after conferring with Leedom, revised his approach. "What I would advise for the jury, if you are concerned, is just close your eyes," Hopper said. "When I see the next slide I will let you know if that is something you should open your eyes for . . . Is that acceptable?"

"These are clinical photographs," Hopper said. "To people not in the medical field, they would be considered potentially gruesome, but they are pictures of a patient in the operating room who has been injured and is undergoing treatment."

Although he explained the procedures matter-of-factly, his descriptions were still horrifying. As Hopper recounted all the details of the initial, fourteen-hour surgery to reconstruct Maria's face, he cataloged the devastation that had occurred. "This entire area should be filled with bone in a human being," he said about her face. ". . . All that bone that should be there is absent . . . If I put my finger right here I would be touching the base of the skull just in front of the spinal cord. So that is how close it was to hitting the spinal cord."

At one point during his testimony a juror announced, "I would like a break."

Hopper's testimony was on the fourth day of what turned out to be a thirty-one-day trial.

Although not necessarily the most technical, Hopper's testimony was the most graphic.

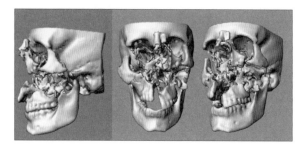

Three dimensional reconstruction of Maria's Harborview CT Scan
Photo admitted as evidence Cause No. 06-02-11563

CHAPTER

33

When Robin listened to the Washington State Patrol's Chief Investigating Detective, Nathan Elias, testify, she was struck all over again with admiration. Along with Anthony Cox and the Medic One crew, he was one of her heroes. Although he came across as incredibly professional, especially now that he was with the FBI, Robin just knew Maria's case had gotten under his skin. If he hadn't put so much effort into the investigation, the driver would probably never have been found, and the link to U-Haul wouldn't have been made. It had all come down to the one witness Elias found, Inge Velde, who had seen Maria's car, the debris, Hefley beside his truck, and the U-Haul open trailer. During his testimony Elias played a video of his interview with Hefley, which showed him denying responsibility for the accident.

Elias, in precise sentences, told the jury about collecting over thirty bags of evidence from a debris trail that was 1,790 feet long, including the palm-sized piece that had been thrown up the embankment. He talked about the witness who saw the U-Haul open trailer. He explained the presence of Hefley's fingerprint on the board that crashed through Maria's windshield, and his U-Haul rental contract for the RO Trailer. Elias stated that Anthony Cox had not seen a vehicle ahead of Maria's Jeep nor had Inge Velde. Elias' conclusions about how the accident occurred would directly refute U-Haul's argument that Maria was partly at fault for following too closely behind

Hefley's vehicle. He stated they were not traveling in the same pack. None of the drivers other than Velde had seen Hefley or the U-Haul trailer.

On October 10, James Hefley testified for the entire day. Robin had seen Hefley outside the courtroom the day before and knew he was "on deck" for the following day. Maria's team had called him an "adverse witness," meaning that his testimony might be prejudiced again the plaintiff's case. Hefley had put on weight since Robin had first seen him. He looked distraught, as if he had suffered since that night. Not in the same way that Maria had suffered, but in the smaller, everyday ways of someone living with regrets. He'd declared bankruptcy. He didn't look healthy or happy. Still, Robin couldn't bear the idea of the jurors watching her face as she watched him, the man who had been transporting the entertainment center that had caused all of the damage to Maria so she stayed away from the courtroom the day he testified. Even if he'd tried his best to fasten the unit, it was still his furniture that had become a weapon.

Even to Maria's attorneys, Hefley didn't seem like a bad person. He came across as just a regular guy who had been driving all weekend, trying to get his new roommate moved from California, and then his stuff moved from his old apartment and friend's garage in Tacoma. As a teenager he'd worked in a lumber yard, so it was established that he was familiar with tying down a load. In February 2004, he was in his late twenties, working as a field technician in telecommunications and moving from south of Seattle to Newcastle, on the east side. His fingerprints were in the system because of what he called "minor issues with the law" when he was young, so he was scared when the police handcuffed and arrested him at work. At first he'd said he had no idea why he was taken in for questioning.

Hefley described driving an enclosed U-Haul trailer from California with a friend's belongings, and then renting the RO Open Trailer on Sunday night for additional moving needs before the enclosed trailer could be unloaded. In his testimony he claimed that he had asked to rent an enclosed trailer but been told they were available only for out-of-state moves. So he rented the RO Open Trailer and proceeded to move a full load of furniture from Tacoma to Newcastle, including a love seat and the entertainment center. After unloading, he and his friend realized that the entertainment center wouldn't fit into the elevator at the new apartment or into the apartment itself. Hefley's friend didn't want the entertainment center so he decided to donate it to the Goodwill. But in the meantime he and his friend loaded it back into the right rear of the open trailer, against the back tailgate where it would be easiest to unload. Hefley's friend then headed for his home in Tacoma, leaving Hefley three ratchet straps to secure the load, plus one that Hefley already had with him.

Hefley decided to take eight to twelve boxes, plus the entertainment center, back to his friend's house in Tacoma to store them again. He said he wasn't aware that Goodwill had twenty-four hour drop-offs. He stacked the boxes and placed one of the two-inch-wide ratchet straps over them, attaching the ends of the straps to rails that ran along both sides of the trailer. Then, according to his testimony, he routed the three remaining ratchet straps over the top of the six-foot-high entertainment center, fastening them to the rails. Each strap went around the rails and then he tightened each one until it was taut. He put the glass doors and entertainment center shelves in the cab of his Dodge Ram and then started on a route that would take him to Interstate 405, southbound.

He testified that he did pull over once on I-405 because he noticed in his driver's side view mirror that a strap was flapping. He said that there wasn't much shoulder there so he was concerned with tying off the strap and then getting off of the roadway. He said that he did not notice that the entertainment center was missing, not until he went to unload it to his friend's garage in Tacoma. He said he was too tired to think through what might have happened to it and never heard any news reports about an object lost on the roadway that night.

As Bill Leedom questioned Hefley he pointed to an almost exact copy of the black entertainment center once owned by Hefley that U-Haul's defense placed in the courtroom. "Do you have any explanation as to how that," pointing at the entertainment center, "got out of the back of the RO trailer, given the description you've provided to the jury as to how you secured it at Newcastle?

"I do not," Hefley replied. "That's something that I think about on a daily basis."

"Why do you do that?" Leedom asked.

"Just the extent of injuries and everything else." Hefley said. "How could you be a part of something like that, indirectly or directly, and not think about that? It's something that's going to haunt me for the rest of my life."

Kleist had a background in war propaganda that made him particularly aware of word choices. He noticed that Leedom and Forgette were using the same words as the defense attorneys, saying Hefley wasn't able to secure his load. "That's bad," Kleist told them. "It puts the blame on Hefley, which is exactly what U-Haul is trying to do. You need to say, 'Hefley was unsuccessful in his attempts to secure his load.'"

But Kleist loved that it was U-Haul that took the jurors down to the loading dock to look at the actual trailer. Forgette and Kleist hung back watching the jurors circle the trailer. It looked even more beat up than when Kleist had rented it two years earlier; it looked like it got battered by objects all the time.

Forgette said to Kleist, "Jesus, that tailgate is low. It looks lower to me every time I see it."

A juror later sent a question through the bailiff, "Why is the tailgate designed so low?" That proved to be one of the questions that U-Haul engineers finally did answer, but it took several weeks.

When the defense presented its case, U-Haul's own witnesses were often vague about the trailer design process, safety testing criteria, and internal communications. In sum, they didn't even defend the engineering of the RO Open Trailer; their position on securing loads was that it was up to the renter.

Robert Dolan, head of the design team for the RO Trailer and a twenty-year U-Haul employee, couldn't confirm that the company had ever conducted a hazards analysis study on its usage; his team did not do any testing on securing loads. Their focus was towards braking with a trailer and whether there was "sway." He denied learning about Maria's incident or any knowledge of other incidents involving the RO Trailer until his subpoena, responding "I didn't learn about it and I did not do any studies to see why. That is someone else's responsibility."

Asked if U-Haul had considered doing safety enhancements to the RO trailer after learning about the twelve accidents this model had been involved in, James Fait, an engineer in U-Haul's test lab, testified, "We looked at claims relative to the number of transactions and when we looked at it percentage-wise–it was just a very, very small number, and it just. . .wasn't getting our attention."

Questioned about a case in which an object had flown out of an RO Trailer, causing a fatality, Fait responded, "Since we don't know exactly what happened in that case we can only come to the conclusion that an item wasn't secured within the trailer to allow it to fall out."

Every witness for U-Haul presented a similar argument: it was never the trailer's fault, it was always the renter. During testimony it emerged that U-Haul didn't even have special instructions for loading the RO Trailer, and whenever changes were made to user's guides, there was no update notice for registered agents and no policy to replace user guides until quantities of older versions were gone. Fait admitted that user guides for trailers didn't include specifics on "load securement," but that supplies were available for sale on the company's website.

Maria's team produced witnesses who demonstrated how RO trailers could be designed more safely and loads secured, for example by providing cargo nets and rings on the bed of the trailer. U-Haul's head of engineering said that cargo nets were never considered because children might be "snarled" up in them. Dolan pointed out the potential for using the side rails on the sides for securing loads, claiming there were an infinite number of places to tie ropes.

As for why the tailgate was so much lower than the side rails, Fait explained it was to deter renters from either driving a backhoe into the trailer or loading the trailer with a backhoe. They wanted the back gate to be too short to form a ramp to the ground to deter such usage. He said it hadn't occurred to the design team that renters might do that until an earlier model had been manufactured, and they realized it "could really bang it up." He reiterated that U-Haul markets its trailers for moving household goods, but their own testing involved cement blocks because the range of what customers might haul was too broad.

A load is either secured, or it isn't, each U-Haul witness testified. Not one of them allowed that there were concerns about the RO trailer or even admitted they had heard of Maria Federici before the lawsuit. Maria's attorneys questioned Dolan about a change to the next model of open six-foot by twelve-foot trailers that added tie-down points to its bed. Why were tie-downs added to the newer HO model but not retrofitted to RO Trailers that were still available for rent? Dolan said there was no need to recall the older RO Trailers because they weren't aware of any problems; he claimed the new tie-downs were due to market demand from motorcycle owners. Dolan also said in response to a question regarding U-Haul's commitment to safety, "I don't know if we have a department that's called safety."

Sitting in the courtroom, Robin was hearing details for the first time about Maria's injuries, the incident investigation, and the management policies of a company that had a location she passed in her car virtually every day. It was overwhelming. As she sat with the attorneys, she wasn't sure how to act in front of the jury; she struggled to control her emotions. It was hard to listen to the defense question witnesses like Mason Blackwell, Maria's supervisor that night. He was such a kind person. He had stayed in touch with Maria and been out to fish with her on the dock. Yet the defense didn't seem want his testimony on how Maria had been driving perfectly in front of him. Instead they hammered on whether he had seen her pour the wine and whether he was familiar with intoxication. Robin felt prepared for how the defense would imply that her daughter should have been in an institution, but she hated to see friends and supporters treated badly.

Strangely, it was an object rather than a person that came to bother her most in the courtroom. She had seen pictures of the board with nails in it that had struck Maria's windshield. She had been told the entertainment center dimensions, but when the defense had a similar model, an "exemplar" as they called it, hauled into the courtroom, she was shocked. It was enormous. From that time on, the jurors had to pass it every time they went to their room. The black object loomed in

Robin's sightline. She couldn't look at it without feeling angry and terribly sad. She thought, how stupid of U-Haul to put this in the courtroom.

On the day of her testimony, Maria's friend, Kristin Shea, or Benecke before her marriage, was waiting in the hallway outside the courtroom. She had agreed to testify as long as Maria wouldn't be present. Talking about Maria in front of her seemed too strange. While she waited, Kristin got to talking to a friendly guy who was also waiting to testify. He was 6'6" to Kristin's 4' 11". Somehow the conversation swung to weddings. The guy was just back from his honeymoon; Kristin was a wedding planner. She felt guilty when she learned he was there as a friend of the driver who loaded the entertainment center onto the trailer with him that night.

Testifying was more difficult than she had imagined it would be. Kristin knew that it was important for the jury to hear about what Maria had been like before the accident, so that they could assess her damages. But Kristin knew the extent of Maria's pride and how much she hated to hear that she was damaged. It felt like a fine balancing act: helping to secure her friend's future meant somewhat betraying her. What Kristin didn't realize until she was on the stand was that Maria's attorneys were using her as an example of what Maria's life could have been like. After all, they'd been to the same schools, received the same degree at the University of Washington, and were just a year apart in age. Kristin felt she represented what Maria would have been doing if she had not been injured. It was surreal for Kristin, very uncomfortable.

Until giving her testimony, Kristin consciously avoided thinking about Maria's injuries and about the Harborview period. She preferred to focus on how much Maria had recovered. What Kristin really wanted to communicate to the jury was: I'm so thankful that Maria is still here. If you look at what she's been able to do since the injury, just think what she could have done without it. She could have done even more because she could do just about anything she put her mind to.

What Kristin had to say when questioned under oath was, "Her recovery is remarkable and I don't want to take that away from Maria, but she is impaired and not the same. . ."

How do you help your best friend without hurting her feelings?

CHAPTER
34

Robin thought Maria's lawyers were doing a great job. Sometimes they kept working at night. On Friday nights Forgette, Kleist, and Pease had pizza together to plan their strategy for the next week—"cuss n'discuss" sessions. Robin believed both Forgette and Leedom were absolute geniuses. Each had his strengths and own rapport with the judge. Judge Hall loved Forgette's ties and had to comment on them each day. Leedom and the judge tended to spar more but Robin could tell the judge thought highly of him. Robin was so proud of all the team: Jan back in the office; Tim Allen, who was simultaneously able to listen and prepare for the next strategic move; and Cate Brewer, who got all the witnesses in and out of town and to the courtroom. She also appreciated the jurors who listened so intently day after day.

Robin felt that Maria's lawyers had strongly conveyed the magnitude of her injuries. They had revealed what seemed to her like arrogance on the part of U-Haul, whose representatives claimed that safety was their number one priority but revealed otherwise.

It was almost time for Robin and Maria to testify. Just as with the deposition, Robin knew that Maria would attempt to paint her life as okay; that was part of her reality. It was Robin's job to present her take on Maria's impairment based on years of daily observation. Judy Maleng had promised to be in the courtroom for Robin on the day of her testimony. They had spoken on the telephone frequently. Strangely enough, Robin wasn't nervous. She had been waiting so long to discuss all that had transpired and all that she had done for Maria's rehabilitation that she felt like she was choking on it. After watching five weeks of testimony from the plaintiff's table, she was more than ready to swear to tell the whole truth as she got to finally face her legal team, her friends Judy Maleng and Heidi Coffee, and strangers who looked kind.

Bill Leedom approached her on the stand. Dear Bill. The golden retriever of her team. "Tell us about the night of February 22, 2004," he said.

Robin took a deep breath and told her story to the court.

Was it curiosity or true concern? Maria was always the one that people wanted to see and hear. Someone from the media had been attending the trial every day, just in case Maria would appear. After hearing so much testimony about her, the jury must have been extremely curious about Maria as well. They had seen more graphic images of her than Robin herself had. What would it be like for the jury to finally meet Maria in person?

The attorneys tried to keep Maria under wraps until the day of her testimony. With such a high profile case, there was always the danger of a mistrial if the jury was tainted by inadvertent media exposure.

Judge Hall had issued orders that allowed only one television camera in the courtroom; it was rolling when Forgette approached Maria in the witness chair.

Forgette had thought for weeks about how best to approach this crucial point of the trial. He couldn't help but think about how they had worked on the case full-time for the last two years, and how it all would culminate with Maria in front of the jury. In truth he'd never had a client who had been so seriously injured but was later able to walk and talk—even testify on her own behalf. He'd decided to consider his questioning of her as more of a conversation.

Forgette first asked what she remembered about the accident and then had her describe her day-to-day life. She spoke of little things that she missed, like tasting and smelling food, being able to open her jaw more than a crack, driving to the store. She answered questions about living with constant headaches and how many times she had broken her toes walking into objects. The jurors submitted questions about her future goals. She responded that she would like to live as normal as a life as would ever be possible. Maria cried as she told about learning that Sammy had been born on the day that she came back to life.

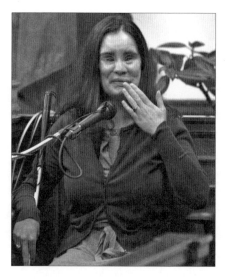

"Maria Federici takes the stand in her case against U-Haul,"
Seattle Post-Intelligencer
Photo by Meryl Schenker Licensed use by Hearst Communications, Inc.

Facing Maria in the witness chair was surprisingly difficult for Forgette. It was probably the most emotional experience he'd ever had in a courtroom. During a break in the testimony, a TV reporter approached Forgette while he was struggling to collect himself. Forgette told him, "Look, I need a couple of minutes." When he'd regained his composure he went to the reporter and said, "Just remember, attorneys don't have feelings."

"Neither do reporters," the broadcaster shot right back.

Maria's testimony was the lead story on the television news that night, and made the front page of both Seattle newspapers the following day.

The morning after Maria's courtroom appearance, the attorneys spent a full hour in discussions with the judge about what questions Tim Allen could ask an engineer from U-Haul. On any given day of the trial, it seemed as if at least an hour was spent arguing over technicalities. When Judge Hall was finally ready to bring in the jury, Capron's attorney, Lisa Marchese, asked her to declare a mistrial on the grounds that the jurors might have been exposed to the news coverage of Maria's testimony. It wasn't the first time the defense had asked for a mistrial, but this time Judge Hall seemed inclined to seriously consider the possibility. She was concerned that Leedom may have improperly discussed the alcohol testing issue with the press. "You need to tell me why this shouldn't be a mistrial," she said directly to Leedom. He explained that he wasn't discussing anything that had not already been public in August.

After a heated discussion, Judge Hall admonished Leedom, then said, "I will now order all parties not to talk to the press." Still concerned as to whether the jurors might have been prejudiced by possible exposure to the coverage, she questioned them one by one. Satisfied that each juror had managed to avoid the news coverage, the judge ordered the trial to continue.

Maria's attorneys couldn't help but notice that of all the alleged engineers and design experts that U-Haul produced, only one witness attempted to defend the RO Trailer, and he didn't even work for U-Haul. His name was Mark Leonard. He had managed to find the entertainment center almost identical to the one Hefley was transporting, strapped it onto an RO Trailer with four ratchet straps, and filmed it being driven around a track to show that it didn't fall off of the trailer. U-Haul played the video for the jury. All of Maria's lawyers noticed something odd about the video. The trailer was being driven on a flat, smooth track and making only left turns. Kleist hoped there were jurors who understood centrifugal force and that on his circuitous route to the freeway Hefley hadn't been able to hold the unit similarly in place. Later in the trial, Leedom and Forgette played U-Haul's video over and over for the jury. Sometimes it seemed like the defense was doing the plaintiff's work.

Kleist had his own theory on how Hefley had lost the entertainment center. He couldn't secure it lying down on the floor of the trailer, so he set it upright in the right rear corner, next to the tailgate, strapped. Each time Hefley came to a stop, momentum would push the unit forward until it worked its way out of the straps, anchored on both sides to side rails that were fifty-five inches below the top of the entertainment center. The straps over the top would have been shaken off as the furniture shifted during hills, turns, and stops. By the time Hefley reached I-405 and attained freeway speed, the top of the unit would have acted like a wing, sending the whole thing flying over the tailgate and into the air.

The sixth and final week of testimony focused on what is called the "damages" portion. Maria's team detailed her medical costs to date, and estimated future medical costs and lost potential earnings based on her projected life span and degree of disability.

U-Haul countered with claims that if Maria's rehabilitation therapy had been more traditional she might be more capable of future employment. They implied she should have been placed in a special facility rather than at home. As for future employment, they proposed the type of work performed by Lighthouse for the Blind employees, or perhaps telephone work.

Maria's attorneys had Copass return to speak as her neurologist about her prognosis and care to date. He explained how the part of her brain injured was responsible for what is known as executive function. Executive function allows a person to apply learned behavior to a present situation. Copass testified that Maria's memory might improve but she could not regain the executive function that would be necessary to take care of herself without aid. Asked about the rehabilitative care she had received at home–the mobility training, voice-activated computer, therapy dog, weight training, and other elements– Copass pronounced Robin's care for her daughter "superb."

Had he ever seen other patients with similar injuries in his thirty years as Harborview's Director of Emergency Services? Copass replied: "I've probably taken care of two dozen individuals who have had this kind of injury and I've never seen one survive; this is the first survivor."

It had been drilled into Robin that there would be one opportunity–and one opportunity only–to make a case against U-Haul. A strange window of time exists in personal injury lawsuits. A patient with a brain injury needs to be at least two years post-injury before doctors can assess prospects for the future. But on the other hand, the statute of limitations for a civil suit–usually three years in cases like this–cannot be reached. Many families know that they cannot survive the years that it takes to get to jury trial, so they end up accepting a settlement instead. Maria was too young for a settlement that might cover just her medical expenses. She had to have money to live on, for she was likely to live for a fairly long time, probably at least another fifty years.

Throughout the trial various representatives approached Maria's lawyers with settlement proposals. None of them was tempting, even when Robin had only a few dollars left in cash. Robin rarely allowed herself to think about losing the case.

It was time for closing statements, after which the case would go to the jury. Forgette and Leedom had argued over which of them would deliver the closing, or summation. They compromised in the way they both felt would best benefit Maria. Leedom did the summation on liability and Forgette spoke to damages.

Pat Schmidt presented the closing argument for the defense. He returned to the themes he had used throughout the trial: U-Haul had provided evidence that the trailer was safe and the company had not been negligent. He expressed sympathy for what had happened to Ms. Federici, but argued that the blame belonged with the driver, James Hefley, and with Maria Federici herself for following too closely, possibly as a result of consuming a glass of wine at the end of her restaurant shift. Leedom, when it was his turn to speak, repeated the assertion that U-Haul was aware of safety issues with the RO Trailers, but chose not to make them safer by equipping them with tie-downs, providing specific safety instructions for open trailers, or even warning customers of the dangers. Forgette, in presenting damages, did not suggest a number for the jury, just a formula they could employ that would help them compensate for each day in her future life that Maria Federici would live with the damages from her injuries.

The case went to the jury on Thursday, November 1.

CHAPTER

35

The judge gave the jury thirty-two pages of instructions and ordered them to appoint a sort of foreperson, called the presiding juror. Dr. Brown, a woman with a PhD degree who worked for the Federal Drug Administration, volunteered and was elected to the role. Based on what she'd heard during the testimony she assumed the verdict would be a slam dunk for the plaintiff based on the facts. Now it was finally time for her peers to deliberate. But that's when things got ugly.

Brown had to admit that the twelve members of the jury (after one alternate was dismissed) represented a pretty accurate cross section of citizens. The testimony had sometimes gone over the heads of one or two of the jurors, particularly the medical testimony and the physics. One of the jurors thought the plaintiff and her mother were simply going after U-Haul because the company had deep pockets. One male juror thought the mother was being overly protective. Others had clearly been listening very thoughtfully and surprised her with their insights. There was a juror who had refused to look at graphic images, and the judge had allowed that. Was it really fair to spare someone from seeing something that might be too disturbing when that was exactly why the lawsuit was brought to trial?

Several jurors thought the plaintiff's attorneys were concealing information about Maria's blood-alcohol, or that the results simply weren't available. Brown listened as some of the jurors engaged in speculation that had nothing to do with the testimony. It was as though they had to get everything out in the open–rid themselves of thoughts and impressions, the emotions and frustrations–that had collected during the six weeks they had not been allowed to speak about them.

Brown didn't share all of her own impressions, unless they were facts. Her background was in epidemiology, public health, and biometrics. She was extremely qualified to weigh all of the medical testimony and the information on product safety. She took notes as allowed so that she could be sure of the details. She felt there had been some real heroes in the events. The bus driver who had stopped at the scene. He was obviously still experiencing post-traumatic stress and could not discuss that night without extreme emotion. He was heroic.

Then there were witnesses who made a poor impression. Defense called to the stand someone Maria had dated, who was also blind. It was clearly inappropriate. He claimed Maria remembered the accident and had confided that she had been drinking. Based on medical facts there was no way that she had any memory connected with the events of that night. It seemed weak on the part of the defense to present an unreliable witness. Plaintiff's attorneys seemed embarrassed as well; they didn't even cross-examine him.

Dr. Brown thought both sides made mistakes, but both sides had strong witnesses as well. The plaintiff's lawyers were able to introduce a few other cases of incidents involving the trailer. Dr. Brown knew enough about corporate insurance to figure that many claims would not even be on record. Their answers about the trailers were evasive. Based on her background analyzing product problems through what are called adverse event reports she knew that whatever is reported is usually just the tip of the iceberg. In her work if there are three reports of product failure, the actual number could be closer to 300.

U-Haul had an engineer testify they had added tie-downs to the trailer in later years because of requests from motorcycle users, which he didn't document. Dr. Brown found that engineer's testimony ridiculous. Maria and her mother's testimony were both very moving. Oddly, what made Maria's testimony moving to Dr. Brown was that it seemed somehow fake. She was obviously a poised, outgoing young woman but her self-perception seemed unrealistic. Her responses seemed too practiced, as though she were acting a role, not as though she'd been coached by the attorneys, but more like a girl playing grown-up. As for Maria's mother, Dr. Brown was inclined to believe her more realistic assessment of the changes in her daughter, beyond the blindness and facial reconstruction. In Ms. Abel's opinion her daughter would never be able to live alone, even though Maria thought she could. Abel gave examples of verbal expressions used incorrectly, childlike behavior and behavioral changes of which her daughter was simply unaware. In response, the defense seemed to want to paint Maria as someone who would be happy and trainable doing menial tasks such as stringing beads. They presented a horrible future presented for her as something she should be happy to attain. In Dr. Brown's assessment, the mother would be looking after her daughter for a very long time.

There was something else besides her impressions that Dr. Brown didn't share with the other jurors. She had been at the wheel of a car struck by a piece of wood that she saw fly out of a garden maintenance truck. It was daylight and she had seen the wood as it went airborne and headed toward her windshield. Unlike Maria's incident, the wood did not come out of no-where–but there was nothing she could have done differently.

The idea of a "slam dunk" evaporated immediately. Jury camaraderie splintered and two distinct "sides" emerged. One side was adamantly opposed to placing any of the blame for the accident on Maria. The other side believed that Maria had been drinking; otherwise she could have avoided the accident. Yet Maria's supervisor had testified that she'd had just one glass of wine. He had driven behind her for miles. Two jurors felt there had been convincing scientific testimony that showed the incident was avoidable. Another faction tended to believe that the accident was entirely Hefley's fault. U-Haul hadn't even been there, why should the company be blamed?

This jury is going to be hung, Brown started to fear. Perhaps unconsciously, she began to do her best to keep that from happening. She knew it had taken years to prepare for the trial, and everyone in the room had been kept from their regular lives since answering the summons months earlier. They had a responsibility to work their way through the jury instructions and the verdict sheet, one decision at a time.

Despite their differences, everyone was trying their best to listen to and show respect for one another. They worked through the questions until they developed a tenuous majority. In discussing the circumstances of that Sunday night so many years ago, they were able to agree that the driver had attempted to secure the contents of the trailer. Quite a few jurors were familiar with his route to the freeway, and it didn't seem likely that the entertainment center would even have gotten to the freeway if it hadn't been secured.

Although a few jurors insisted it was easy to know how to load a trailer, most did not. Telling renters that they could go to a store to buy rope didn't strike the jurors as particularly safety-conscious. Plus, everyone had to admit that the design of the trailer was odd, with its low sides and even lower tailgate.

The jurors discussed what constituted a hung jury. No one wanted to be the one to tell the judge they couldn't reach a decision. They respected Judge Hall. "We need ten people to agree on each count," Brown reminded them before they each voted. Brown felt it was her responsibility as presiding juror to help everyone feel safe about the decisions they were making together. Taking it one question at a time helped to simplify the process. It was easier to break the issues down this way, and slowly they moved toward consensus.

After a week of discussion, the jury reached a decision. It was Friday, November 9. "Let's call the bailiff," Brown said.

When the bailiff received the news that the jury had reached a verdict, he called both sets of attorneys and members of the local news media. He gave them only about half an hour to get to the courthouse. In Kirkland, Forgette, Pease, and Kleist tried not to behave like the Three Stooges as they rushed for the car.

"I can't get there," Robin said rather flatly when Forgette called her, as though not allowing herself the emotion of hope. Earlier that day she had driven to the other side of Puget Sound to visit what proved to be her Grandmother Kitty's deathbed. Robin had held her hand while telling her, "Maria is going to be okay. It's all right to let go." Just before Simon's call she received the phone call from her mother that Grandma had died without regaining consciousness. Robin and Forgette had discussed beforehand whether she and Maria should try to get to the courtroom for the verdict, but it would be impossible this late on a rainy Friday. Robin did not want herself or Maria to have to hear the verdict while being watched by the media. It was one of the few times she allowed herself to picture the wrong outcome.

"We'll call you the minute that we've heard," Forgette promised.

Judy Maleng just happened to be near downtown Seattle when she heard on the radio that the Federici jury had reached a verdict. She had been looking forward to getting home until she heard the news. Judy knew that she had to be in the courtroom, especially because she doubted that Robin could get there on such short notice from her home in the country. She parked her car and took the elevator up to the ninth floor of the courthouse. She watched all the attorneys arrive, along with the throngs of media people, some of whom she recognized. Then the bailiff announced the arrival of the judge, who brought in the jury. Judy knew that Robin had been focused for years on her daughter, and that she and Maria were living on a shoestring. As she sat waiting for the announcement, Judy concentrated her thoughts on a verdict that would be a win for Robin and her daughter.

Judge Hall read the verdict rather than the presiding juror. Patty Pease, Forgette's assistant, held her breath until she heard the words, "Jury finds plaintiff has no liability." Oh, thank heavens, she thought. We need to call Robin. Forgette pulled out his cell phone.

"We won," Forgette whispered to Robin. "We won."

The jury assigned sixty-seven percent of the liability to U-Haul International and U-Haul Washington, and thirty-three percent to the driver. They found U-Haul and Hefley negligent and liable, with Capron Holdings negligent but not liable.

After Forgette's phone call, Robin's phone rang again immediately. "Yes, Simon," she almost said.

"Robin, it's Kathi Goertzen."

"Kathi! I just this second heard from the attorney. How could you find out so quickly?"

Goertzen laughed, "Well, I am the media. Can we come out and see you?

Robin knew Goertzen really cared about her and Maria. She'd never forgotten her help getting the second bill passed. So it was Goertzen's KOMO-News 4 that earned the exclusive interview with Robin and Maria on the 11:00 p.m. news that night. Maria told Goertzen, "It [the verdict] was a complete relief. It really was. I can have a house, a place to live. And just try to pick up where I left off three-and-a-half years ago. And just live and spend time with my friends and just do the same things that I always used to do."

Robin said she was happy but so emotionally drained that she could barely think. The jury verdict called for $15.5 million. Robin knew the ordeal wasn't over yet. Goertzen ended the KOMO piece with these sobering words: "U-Haul said they planned to appeal Friday's decision. Federici's lawyer said they are prepared to fight the case to the end."

Forgette and the rest of the legal team allowed themselves a weekend to celebrate, while Robin and Maria attended Grandma Kitty's funeral.

CHAPTER

36

"Woman blinded on I-405 gets $16 million" blazed the headline in the Seattle Post-Intelligencer the day after the verdict, but in reality Maria didn't have a dollar more than she had had a month earlier. A jury verdict is not like winning the lottery. There's no presentation of an oversized check. Instead, despite the verdict, Robin was forced to calculate how long they could survive on the money they had left. Maria still qualified for medical aid from the state. Robin figured they could live for a few years with what money remained from the fundraisers, but she hoped they didn't have to do that.

The appeal process is a gamble; a judge can always overturn a verdict and any chance of receiving a settlement can be lost. The appeal process is also expensive; transcribing even portions of the trial can cost thousands of dollars. Speaking to reporters immediately after the verdict, one of U-Haul's lawyers had the nerve to bring up the blood-alcohol test again, saying that it should have been admitted as evidence. When Robin read that, she wanted to shout, what about the incidents involving other trailers (the judge had permitted the jury to hear only about eleven others specific to RO trailers) that our side wasn't allowed to use?

Forgette and Leedom told her they needed to decide whether to dispute U-Haul's grounds for appeal, and in turn specify what parts of the trial they wanted to use for their argument. Then U-Haul let a deadline pass for filing a specific request. In the meantime Forgette kept calling U-Haul's insurance representative regularly, "Let's try to get together on this one more time." Whenever Forgette was in New York City on business he would drop in personally with the insurance adjustor; finally something came of the prodding.

Even without a settlement, Robin had decided that if they won the court case they could at least make another step towards Maria's independence. The cabin just next door was unoccupied and Robin talked to the owner about renting it to Maria starting in December. It was close enough for Robin to watch out for Maria. Maria still had a caregiver during the day. When Maria moved next door Robin listened and worried but she was very proud of Maria's progress.

The fourth anniversary of Maria's accident, or "incident," as Robin had long trained herself to say, came and went. Robin resumed her efforts to promote safety now that it was no longer something that U-Haul could use against her at the trial. At this point any speaking honoraria were needed to pay bills— even though Robin would never turn down an opportunity just because a group couldn't pay. Although most of the public probably thought her daughter was rich now, they had never been more short of funds. Six months after the verdict, a representative from U-Haul and its insurer finally said yes to sitting down with a mediator.

"Tell yourself it's going to be your lucky day," Judy Maleng told Robin by phone on the morning of the mediation. "Buy a lottery ticket."

"It's our lucky day," Robin told Maria and the attorneys when they met downtown. At first they didn't seem to want her to get her hopes too high, but then they seemed to start sharing her good mood.

The mediation process can take place in many different arenas, between divorcing parents who have custody issues, between business partners who need help dividing their assets, and between legal parties who must weigh the lengthy appeal process against the prospect of moving on. The two parties are in separate rooms; the mediator goes back and forth between them. Offers are proffered, then countered. Points are raised, then agreed upon or eliminated. Depending on the terms of the settlement, records can be sealed, award amounts can be confidential.

The mediation started in the morning and continued until afternoon. Robin had always had a figure in mind that she hoped would be enough to sustain Maria for the rest of her life. By late in the afternoon, an offer was placed on the table that Robin and Maria could accept.

Leedom typed up the agreement himself, as there was no time to delegate the task. The amount on the table would have to cover attorney fees, and was less than the verdict headlines would have one believe. In addition, part of the settlement money would reimburse Medicaid for Maria's care and Robin for some of her out-of-pocket expenses over the past years. But all that really mattered was that it would be enough for Maria to be able to live independently.

Robin drove home to Lake Kathleen still just wishing that she had never received that horrendous phone call from Harborview in the first place. If this part was supposed to be justice, it was hollow. Norm Maleng had said justice isn't always about winning. True, she thought, we won, we finally have agreement on a dollar amount, but it was just another day, and nothing could restore what had been lost. It wasn't as if U-Haul had agreed to change their safety practices or Maria would ever regain her sight.

Life didn't change. Spring turned to summer. The garden flourished. The dogs romped. Maria continued to ask friends to describe exactly what was pictured in fashion magazines and still loved to talk about food, even if she couldn't enjoy eating it. She lived very much in the moment, discussing future career plans but not yet pursuing them. Her headaches became simply a way of life. She liked keeping her things orderly in her own space next door.

Robin was at the vet's office with her oldest golden retriever, Beau, the one that Maria had brought home in Utah, when Bill Leedom called her cell phone. "We've got it," he said. "The check arrived!"

Robin started to cry from sheer relief. It was really over now. Four years from when she'd retained Forgette, there was a resolution. "That's great news," she said. "That's great."

She hung up and saw Dr. Jackson, the vet, waiting for her to finish the call. Jackson shook her head. "No," she said simply: Beau couldn't be treated. Robin stroked Beau while Dr. Jackson administered the lethal injection, her tears dropping onto Beau's still-gorgeous coat.

Robin drove home alone to tell Maria about Beau. The night that Maria's financial future was resolved, they cried together over the death of a beloved dog. Robin thought about how most people would think it strange that they would be sobbing and not rejoicing over the money. It's just money, Robin thought. We would both give back every single penny to go back to the moment before the board went through Maria's windshield. Every penny.

A month after the final check was issued by the insurers, that company's potential collapse sent the international and domestic economy reeling. "Robin must have someone watching over her," Simon's paralegal Patty Pease said.

That fall Maria and varying family members went house-hunting with Maria. They would visit open houses to see if the house could fit Maria's specific mobility needs. While most of the family moved between neighborhoods in a caravan of cars,

Bobby insisted on bicycling. He was assessing the bus routes, the curb cuts, the proximity of a grocery store and a park for walking the dogs.

On a Thursday in October 2008, Maria moved to her own newly purchased home. She took almost nothing except her clothes, her dogs, and items from her old apartment that had been in storage. Mostly she wanted to start fresh with new furniture, new things. After Maria left, Robin stood outside the cabin looking toward the empty road, her golden retrievers nudging against her legs as if they knew she needed comfort. Robin had done everything in her power, and sometimes beyond, to rebuild her daughter's life. Now, for the second time, her daughter had left the nest the way that all children are meant to leave when they are ready.

Robin still sometimes dreams of the childhood Maria. She will always miss her daughter—the fearless girl she raised and the amazing one who was given back to her after the accident. Robin started her campaign for road safety because of Maria—but now it is for everyone.

AFTERWORD

"I've been through five legislative sessions but I can count on one hand, minus one finger, how many times bills have made it through the process because a family member was determined to have something good come out of a tragedy."

Governor Christine Gregoire, July 29, 2009

If Maria's accident began like a movie, it eventually became an epic film, one with a cast of thousands, from the Washington State Patrol to the social workers, from everyone who sent a card or flowers, to the scale operators at transfer stations, ferry workers, and the hundreds of people who donated so much as spare change "for Maria." Six years later no one has forgotten. Everyone remains haunted by the photo that ran for so many days while State Patrol appealed for information. They think of Maria Federici when they see an unsecured couch in the back of a truck, debris in their lane on the Interstate, or hear about teenagers throwing stones from overpasses. "I wonder how Maria is doing," strangers often wonder.

Every time there's an incident involving road debris, the media shares Maria's story. Her name and "Maria's Law" have come to represent all such incidents. When people spend an extra ten minutes tying down their load before driving to the transfer station, they "do it for Maria." Each person has a story about an encounter or near-miss with road debris–from the Chief of the Washington State Patrol, John Batiste, to Robin's mother.

No one has forgotten.

Now living in her own home, Maria has a life that revolves around her dogs. In addition to her first Cavalier, Sammy, she has a female, Sadie Mae. Then there is Nick, an older rescue dog. Even as Maria continues to improve, medical issues remain. Debris imbedded in her face that night in February, 2004, still works its way close to the surface of her skin and needs to be surgically removed: a piece of metal, a shard of glass.

Maria still loves to shop and talk about fashion. She calls her mother often to exchange dog stories. Every few weeks they go out to lunch even though Maria has mostly lost her sense of taste. For Maria's thirtieth birthday Robin arranged for Kerri, younger sister of Maria's friend Kristen, to be their personal shopper at Nordstrom. Maria's memory loss has never included Nordstrom.

"Can Maria see?" people ask Robin when they learn that she is Maria's mom. She considers the question a tribute to the artistry of the two women who crafted Maria's prosthetic brown eyes. "Maria cannot see," Robin answers, but even that seems inaccurate. She has no vision but only Maria knows what she can see in her mind's eye: what she pictures when a friend describes each accessory in a fashion magazine, what plays in her mind when she hears a story about herself as a child. Can she remember how her dog Arthur looked up at her as the school bus pulled away? Does she remember her mother's face as it was before the accident? Maria cannot see the lines etched on her mother's face by pain and sleeplessness over the last six years.

Beginning with the moment of impact, Maria's life changed in an instant. Even as her new face healed, her belongings were packed into a storage unit, and her apartment was rented to someone else. Five months after the accident the Washington State Patrol released her car. Local dealerships donated parts and labor for its repair and then Wells Fargo picked up the car and wrote off the remaining debt. Maria will never be able to drive again but her former car is probably still on the road somewhere–even though U-Haul's defense referred to the Jeep Liberty as "evidence that had been destroyed."

Maria bought all new furniture for her new home, which she made sure had lots of closets so that she could organize things exactly as desired. She chose a neighborhood that was pedestrian-friendly for her and her beloved dogs. Just before her thirtieth birthday, Maria did something she had wanted to do since the days of playing travel agency with her cousin Kristina. Maria visited Italy for the first time–after all, her last name is Federici and her favorite food is pasta.

Maria's greatest desire is to live as normal a life as possible. She comments if the media contacts her about incidents involving road debris, but it is not her mission. She texts with friends and family and calls her grandparents, but she doesn't socialize as much as she did when she was younger. Maria leads a comparatively quiet life.

For the people who became players in the Federici story, scars remain.

Anthony Cox the Metro bus driver who stopped that night and saved Maria's life, finds the incident too painful to discuss. Jean Gamboa still replays the moment, even as she makes the same commute she did six years ago. One of the Renton firefighters who removed Maria from her car at the scene and tried to give her oxygen has just graduated from the Medic One program, inspired by watching Medic One save Maria's life that night.

Dr. Michael Copass stepped away from day-to-day responsibility for Emergency Services at Harborview after thirty years, but is still highly involved with the facility, Medic One, and his neurology clinic. At a Medic One fundraiser, he and Jim Stevens discussed the Federici case. "Who got in the trach?" he asked the paramedic. "My partner," Stevens replied. "It was a one-in-a-million chance," Copass told him.

King County Executive Ron Sims was tapped by the Obama Administration to be Deputy Secretary for Housing and Urban Development in Washington, D.C. With regard to tragedies such as happened to Maria he said, "I wish there could be a law against stupidity." He doesn't believe people are being malicious when they don't secure their loads, just ignorant of the danger.

Dan Satterberg was elected King County's Prosecuting Attorney a few months after Norm's death. He remembers the events surrounding the incident and legislation quite well, commenting, "The Maria Federici story is really the Robin Abel story." He was Norm's Chief of Staff for seventeen years; he and Judy Maleng remain close. Judy Maleng and Robin Abel once attended his daughter's school play; he never knows when they may turn up together.

The law firm of Bennett, Bigelow & Leedom has continued with mostly defense work, but their plaintiff work on behalf of Maria is still a great source of pride. Bill Leedom has a daughter exactly the same age as Maria, so the case was always somewhat personal; it stands as one of the biggest damage awards he has helped a client attain. But Bill Leedom still thinks the damages should have been higher. As years pass and memory of the excruciating week in Arizona trying to get information from U-Haul fades, Tim Allen, the former debate coach, still looks back on the case as "fun," because the adversaries were worthy and the outcome was what they had hoped.

Bennett, Bigelow & Leedom paralegal Cate Brewer knows the Federici case is one that will stay with her forever. For a period of six months before the trial she worked ten hours a day, six days a week going through virtually every piece of paper associated with the case. It would have been a page-turner for any law firm but mysteries about the case still fascinate her. How did Maria's car travel almost 2,000 feet after she was struck? What miracle brought it to rest beside the divider? Cate drives the same stretch of Interstate 405 and thinks, Maria is so lucky to be alive, and to be able to have a life that she's enjoying.

Everyone who has been with Simon Forgette "forever" is still there–Jan Nevler, Patty Pease, Denise Weldon, and Carol Hodovance. After the settlement, Simon put together a memorandum for colleagues in which he shared some of the facts about the Federici case that were never reported in the media. He found it particularly frustrating that the media reported U-Haul's suggestion that Maria was drunk at the time of the accident, but never refuted this claim. Once Simon put those issues on paper, he claimed to stop thinking about the case, but he can recount the details readily. Everyone in his office is proud of what they have accomplished using tort law to get companies to change for the sake of the consumer.

Murray Kleist let his license to practice law expire after the Federici case, claiming there just was not another big one to draw him back. Simon still lists him as consultant on the web site because Murray can always be coaxed to offer at least an opinion. The outcome of the Federici trial remains one of their biggest wins; the verdict represents one of the largest recoveries in a personal injury case in state history.

The Honorable Judge Glenna Hall left the bench at King County Superior Court the summer after the Federici case. It was her biggest final case. She moved to San Juan Island where she still serves as judge pro tem as well as providing mediation services. It surprises her still how well-known the Federici versus U-Haul trial continues to be; new colleagues always comment when they learn she was the judge. She is confident she made the right decision in excluding the ETOH test from

Harborview. When the jury was out for so long, she worried there would be a mistrial, but she looks back on the case as well argued by both sides. "They were all very good lawyers, which makes a judge's job easier." The trial also stands as the only time a juror asked her to perform a wedding ceremony. When she walked into the courtroom and saw the Federici jurors back in their assigned jury seats for the wedding vows she was flabbergasted. She was honored to be asked to perform the ceremony and she's glad she did it.

Although it has been over two years since the Federici trial, the presiding juror, Dr. Brown, still thinks about the case. The trial was not something she expected in her life, but she's come to believe that she was meant to be on that jury. Along with some of the other jurors she wishes the damages award could have been higher. Maria's whole life had been altered at the age of twenty-four; that was really very, very young. It wasn't until after she went home that Friday that she learned just how much media attention had been focused on the case, and on Maria, dating back for years. She went to her computer and started looking back at what had been written. It made her angry to learn that the driver had had a suspended license and no car insurance. She'd felt all along that the gas station where Hefley had rented the trailer bore some responsibility for the incident. The station had just taken his money and made a profit on the deal. As for U-Haul, she sensed they were stonewalling on the stand, trying to act like their trailer was not a factor. Why couldn't they just be a good corporate citizen? The trailer was potentially dangerous.

Dr. Brown was certain, based on her background in analyzing product problems, that the industry had been alerted to the dangers – but they put horse's ass engineers on the stand who adamantly refused to accept responsibility. Why fight it to the bitter end? Why not do the right thing and make trailers that performed safely? When Dr. Brown sees an open U-Haul trailer, she notices whether the back gate is higher than the one in the accident, whether there are tie-downs. On her commute she drives a similar route through Bellevue that Hefley had taken. One day she saw a U-Haul truck that couldn't make it up the hill because its load had shifted to the back of the vehicle. They'd put wedges under the tires and were trying to shift the load closer to the cab. Had anyone told them how to load the truck, she wondered? Was it another case of a teenager renting out equipment without instructions?

There is no evidence that U-Haul ever recalled the RO Open Trailer to be retrofitted with interior tie-downs. But as of 2004 U-Haul began producing the HO model with a higher back tailgate and interior tie-downs. It's impossible to say when this wording appeared but the Open Trailers section on U-Haul's website now references the possibility that, "Cargo not properly secured may shift, be damaged or be ejected under normal driving conditions." The section also now includes the phrase, "Secure your load, it's the law."

After Norm's death, Judy Maleng continued to hear from programs and agencies wanting to pay tribute to Norm. She and her son Mark discussed how the recognition would have embarrassed Norm, but they came to realize the sincerity of each honor. "Funerals are for the living," Norm had told his son; they realized they could not deny the rights of others to pay tribute. Judy and Mark continue to witness the long-term impacts of Norm's contributions—creating the domestic violence unit, drug court, a program of therapy dogs for child victims.

The year after Norm's death, Judy and Mark went to the dedication of the Norm Maleng Building at Harborview Medical Center. They had a private tour several days in advance of the ribbon-cutting. The new building was beautiful. Instead of claustrophobic waiting rooms for the families of patients, a sky bridge faced Mount Rainier with reclining chairs. The building had state-of-the-art design for trauma patients and five additional operating rooms. The corridors were filled with artwork and sculptures. On a chilly June day Judy and Mark Maleng used oversized scissors to cut the ceremonial ribbon in front of the door to the new building. Later there would an even bigger dedication when King County decided to rename the Regional Justice Center in Norm Maleng's honor. But for Judy the Harborview connection is the one that really speaks to his professional and his personal commitment.

Robin's parents, Bob and JoRene, continue to divide their time between Las Vegas and a cabin on Wollochet Bay. JoRene joined an organization in Las Vegas called Blind Connect that provided mentors to teach about issues facing the blind. They are proud of all of their children, but what strikes them about Robin is how the child who once nursed an injured crow in her bedroom has become such a powerful "Mama Bear" on issues of road safety. As for Maria, they love her spirit, the fact that she never complains about what happened and is always so upbeat. They just want their first-born grandchild to have all the happiness she deserves.

Robin's sisters love to shop with Maria and celebrate birthdays. Robin's brother Bobby still insists on bicycling everywhere–to Seattle during a snowstorm, to the Olympic Peninsula for a professional conference. He went through a withdrawal when he stopped visiting Robin and Maria every single week. It was hard for him to stop being so much a part of their lives. His wife Kim is no longer the mayor of Port Orchard but is applying her political experience and law degree to help Robin draft national legislation on securing loads. "Secure Your Load" may not be Maria's passion, but changing people's behavior has become Robin's life work.

Maria's childhood best friend, Kristin Shea, is back working in the same location in Seattle, the Sorrento Hotel, from where she could walk to Harborview after work every day. When she and Maria get together, she relishes Maria's trademark sarcasm. She's known both Maria and Robin since she was a kid and reflects, "I wouldn't have guessed that either one of them would turn out to be as much of a fighter."

All of Robin's safety contacts continue to be her foot soldiers even as government agencies struggle to keep anti-litter campaigns and emphasis patrol grants in their budgets. They have accomplished many goals together since "Maria's Law" first went into effect. "Secure Your Load" signs are posted at transfer stations all over the state. The Driver's License booklet and test include references to the law. There have been bus and radio ads, brochures, educational videos for citizens and commercial drivers, lighted highway signs, and speeches all over the state of Washington. "Maria's Law" was only the first step.

Robert Ott, who secured Maria's first computer system for the blind, has served on the Maria Federici Foundation board since its inception. Heidi Coffee, Gavin's widow, is new to the board. She is also working towards a law degree. Therese Sangster and Lisa Rios, Maria's Medusa co-workers who were instrumental organizing the largest fundraiser, are also board members, Therese since the very beginning. And Therese married the handsome man who delivered the signed Pearl Jam guitar to the fundraiser in the nick of time.

After Maria moved to her own home, Robin experienced something akin to combat fatigue. For five years she had been fighting battles on so many fronts it was as if the sudden end was deafening. She had been listening for Maria acutely ever since the return to Harborview. Listening for her first words, her moaning, her movements in the night, her first steps on her own, the first trip to the mailbox, listening for any problems when she moved to the cabin next door–Robin had been listening for years. Yet she found she didn't much care for silence right after Maria left.

Over the course of five years, she had not had even ten days away from Maria. At first there were the weeks at Harborview, and once Maria was home, her times away were carefully measured, like elementary school recesses. Days at court during the seven weeks of the trial had been her longest time away from Maria for all those years, throughout surgeries and clinic visits, the trips to Olympia. After Maria left home for the second time, Robin found that she just wanted to sink into a soft chair and cocoon herself in one of the heirloom quilts she had discovered at a Goodwill store. She didn't want to cook; she certainly didn't want to eat. If she had been able to sleep, she would have liked to catch up on what seemed like years of interrupted slumber.

Her dormant period didn't last long. Even while she felt as though she were choking on all that had happened, Robin needed to start physically and mentally shoveling the experience out of her. She began to organize her memories of everything that had happened, beginning with that first urgent phone call from Harborview.

Then she switched gears and ordered literally tons of dirt. If she could find energy for anything, it was for her garden. Once again, Robin began digging and planning, digging and planning. She started walking around the lake again each morning, but she added another element to her walk by collecting litter every single day–the least she could do for her neighbors and for Megan Warfield.

After Maria left, Robin's golden retriever Sky became even more attached to her, as though trying to fill the void. One day, a new idea came to Robin as Sky helped her retrieve litter along the roadside. She would have a vest made for Sky to wear to speeches and safety conferences–bright orange, the color of safety. Sky would be her ambassador wearing her specially made "Secure Your Load" vest. Who could resist a dog?

Robin had always planned to go national with legislation as part of her own four-part plan. Get Maria well, get a law established in Washington State, secure Maria's future, and then take the bill national. She began to call everyone who had ever promised to help, anyone she thought could help. Robin arranged meetings with Chief John Batiste of the Washington State Patrol, and King County Sheriff Sue Rahr–everyone agreed with what she had to say: legislation for Secure Your Load should be national because it would save lives.

On one of the hottest days on record in Washington State, Robin was ushered back to Chris Gregoire's office, but the Capitol building was cool like the Governor's white loveseats. "I want to make "Maria's Law" national," Robin blurted out to Chris Gregoire, nervousness overcoming her thought-out remarks.

"And you should," the Governor replied, catching Robin off guard with her immediate support.

"A lot of people think it's foolish to try," Robin said.

"I don't agree," Gregoire said. "These incidents could be preventable." Robin was momentarily confused when Chris Gregoire said, "I'll give Patty and Maria a call…" She was talking about U.S. Senators Patty Murray and Maria Cantwell. "I can probably make a personal call to someone on the House side as well."

Robin sat there wondering even as she and Chris Gregoire continued to talk, had the Governor really just offered to make phone calls on behalf of national legislation?

"It's the human piece of the job that gives you the satisfaction," Gregoire told Robin when she walked Robin out to the antechamber."As the mom of two daughters I'm so grateful for your work on this." Once again she extended her hand for a firm handshake and squeeze.

Robin felt more fully alive after the meeting with Gregoire than she had felt since the accident, almost too excited to drive. Although Robin was not usually one for symbolism, she had come to associate butterflies with rebirth and transformation. It still made her smile to remember Maria when she was in the Rehab unit linking the words, peanut butter and butterflies. All these last years she had been thinking that Maria was the one being transformed, going through metamorphosis to emerge like one of their beautiful Lake Kathleen butterflies. Robin realized that she too had been transformed, made stronger by her daughter's miraculous recovery. Robin would ask her sister-in-law Kim Abel to draft the legislation. Even if it took every ounce of nerve, she would cold-call families that had lost someone to road debris in other states. Robin would drive across the country if need be, state by state, to gain support for legislation.

She would never forget the phone call that had come out of nowhere to shatter their lives, but Robin allowed herself to picture the signing day on national legislation that could prevent other incidents; she hoped that Maria would be at her side. If only the process didn't take so long; what about the deaths and injuries that could occur before a Secure Your Load law was enacted across the country? This is what I was meant to do because Maria survived, Robin thought, and it's for those who didn't.

On Friday, December 4, 2009 there was a three-car accident in the early afternoon on a New York City expressway. An SUV swerved to avoid cable wire in the right lane, sending a semi-truck belonging to the United States Postal Service into the far left lane, into the path of a third vehicle. The twenty-eight year old woman driver of the SUV was thrown to her death some seventy feet below the expressway. Her name was Suejas Estrada. Her co-workers at a car dispatch service overheard radio calls for emergency response without knowing the victim was their colleague. The driver of the postal truck had minor injuries and the third car had only damages.

The incident wasn't national news because of a young woman's death, but because the third car was driven by NBC News anchorman Tom Brokaw, who along with his wife Meredith, was uninjured. Law enforcement issued a statement that although the accident appeared to be caused by debris there was "no criminality involved."

Robin Abel would beg to differ. Unlike Maria, Suejas Estrada did not survive. Robin Abel will not allow that to be the end of another young woman's story.

ACKNOWLEDGMENTS

This book is a tribute to everyone who opened their hearts to Maria and me since the night of February 22, 2004, including unknown well wishers across the globe. Still I have to name some of the friends, strangers and professionals who have been real life angels over the years.

Thank you to Anthony and Jean who stopped for Maria that night; they are my first two heroes. Without Inge Velde the truth about what happened might never have been known. Heartfelt thanks to Renton Fire Department and Medic One. Without Dr. Michael Copass at Harborview Medical Center Maria wouldn't be alive today because he personally trained and directed Medic One. His trained staff in Emergency Services pulled out every stop to save Maria.

Dr. Richard Hopper, her plastic surgeon, is a wizard and an artist; his team's work to reconstruct Maria's face was nothing short of miraculous. His Surgical Fellow Dr. Anna Kuang was the first to give me hope with her smile and positive attitude. Also at Harborview, Dr. Amadi looked after Maria's eyes, Dr. Ellenbogen was lead neurosurgeon. Dr. Kaufman and the Speech Therapist Ross in the Rehabilitation Unit were terrific. But among the everyday heroes at Harborview are Karen at the front desk, Jon in Intensive Care and Sydney Ho who navigated us through financial assistance. Maria's dentist Dr. Vendeland and his staff fixed Maria's teeth and did everything in her mouth for free for several years. The "Seattle Eye Gals" Rebecca Erickson and Amy Wellner at Erickson Laboratories exhibited artistry in making Maria's ocular prosthetics, giving her big, beautiful brown eyes again.

I wish *Out of Nowhere* could do greater justice to the genius and tenacity of our legal "Dream Team." Simon Forgette, the team leader, always made me feel safe with his wisdom and quiet strength. Jan Nevler, his associate, reviewed hundreds of documents with keen eyes yet always held my hand. Without Murray Kleist there might not have been a trial at all. With their defense experience and medical background Bill Leedom, Tim Allen and Cate Brewer at Bennett, Bigelow & Leedom completed the team. Bill Leedom is not only brilliant but funny. He has a special finesse; the courtroom is like a dance to him and he doesn't miss a beat. Tim was the "Brief King," responding immediately to nearly one hundred motions. Cate was invaluable in trial preparation and in support of this book. Simon and Bill were the ultimate warriors in the courtroom on behalf of Maria and public safety.

Thank you to the jury, including the alternate sent home after testimony but still on-call through deliberations. These citizens were truly everyday heroes who sacrificed months of their lives performing their civic duty with honor.

Thank you to all the media; their support helped locate the driver, brought people to the fundraisers, built support for the legislation and provided public service in communicating the importance of road safety. They have treated us with amazing respect. Very special thanks to Kathi Goertzen for her kindness and professionalism. ("You are a class act".) Peter Alexander, now of NBC, was an outstanding emcee at the fundraiser, his continued interest in our welfare and his prompt responses mean the world to me. Deborah Feldman and Molly Shen also deserve acknowledgment. Thank you to local columnists Robert Jamieson Jr., Mary Swift and Mike Archbold and so many other reporters who all sincerely cared about Maria.

Norm Maleng continues to be my guardian angel. As a state senator said during legislation, "You couldn't have a better one." Thank you to Judy Maleng who has listened to me cry so often–and fulfilled her promise of "being there" for me. Prosecuting Attorney Dan Satterberg and his Chief of Staff Leesa Manion have given me strength through their ongoing support for legislation and victims rights. King County under the leadership of Executive Ron Sims made Secure Your Load a priority within all departments, acting as a model for other counties in Washington State.

Then there are the safety warriors from various government and private organizations: Megan Warfield, Layne Nakagawa, Polly Young, Tom Odegaard, Ric Gleason, Ray Clouatre, John Carlson, Milo Pipkin, Tony Gomez, Mike Southards and Char Alexander with the Governor's Annual Health & Safety Conference. I also need to thank Lowell Porter and Steve Lind of the Washington Traffic Safety Commission for their support and grant funding. Thank you to those on the front lines–the scale operators.

I am grateful to Sherry Palmiter for her incredible support building and managing a web site after Maria's incident. Her role as Board Member of the original foundation was huge. All of my Board Members – friends and acquaintances are all foot soldiers for the cause. I don't know where I would be without original members Carole Kirkpatrick, Dan Pollack, Robert Ott, Krysten Cook, and Therese Sangster, plus newer members Lisa Rios and Heidi Coffee.

To Peter Kissinger, President of AAA National Organization – Your words of encouragement kept me giong!

Thank you to my friends John Petrie and Gary Abrahams who both acted as "legal quarterbacks" at different stages.

I'll never forget the emotional generosity of those who organized fundraisers: everyone who put together the fundraiser at Medusa, Richard Geiler, the Kings of Swing, my former classmates at Chief Sealth, those who collected at their place of business, and of course Don & Loretta Stevenson. Thank you to everyone who contributed to their events.

I couldn't have survived financially without help from my parents Bob and JoRene who didn't charge me any house payments so that I could afford to be home with Maria. To my family who could not have provided any more support in the world during three months in the hospital. They dropped everything to help and their support continues. My sister-in-law Kim Abel just drafted national legislation.

I need to thank the Gavin Coffee family, Babe Watson, Dawn Jacobs and all of the families and victims of unsecured loads and brain injury who let me into their lives.

The Washington State Patrol and the King County Sheriff have been incredibly supportive from initial investigation through every emphasis patrol. Thank you to Chief John Batiste and Sheriff Sue Rahr.

Kate Dussault and The Dussault Law Group–Kate, you are an angel to me. You made sense of the state's paperwork and simplified the process for me. Without someone like you how would the average person work through the system I call, "A maze with no cheese."

Thank you to all my neighbors around the lake...Faye Moss and the Moss family, Sherry, Greg and Adam, Diane and Gary, Joan and Cliff. Thank you Marcia Berenter for your guidance and friendship. I have to especially thank Howard and Robin for all the wonderful floating dock excursions, gourmet meals and campfire talks. Maria and I were honored to spend time with the seven guide dogs that you have raised. Lastly, Howard–when I asked you about writing a book, your advice was to just do it. Well Howard, here it is.

Bless all of Maria's caregivers because each one was fabulous. Caregivers are underappreciated, underpaid and yet desperately needed. Thank you to Maria's personal trainer Tracy Morales and to Diane Rich, Maria and Sammy's therapy dog trainer.

Thank you to Maria's wonderful friends who showed maturity beyond their years, including her supervisor the night of the incident, Mason Blackwell.

In Olympia, thank you to Ruth Kagi for sponsoring "Maria's Law" in the House. Sincere thanks to Governor Christine Gregoire for making an ordinary person feel special.

Finally, thank you to Maria for showing me the way to courage. You are my inspiration.

Peggy Sturdivant wants to acknowledge everyone who participated in personal interviews and provided source materials for this book. Special thanks to Judy Maleng for her contributions to the entire process; her forthrightness shaped my work. The Washington Law Review article of February 2009, "The Legacy of Norm Maleng" by Robert S. Lasnik and David Boerner provided an excellent overview of Norm's career.

Thank you to Scott McCredie for his counsel and editing, Lee Schoentrup and Mary Fickes for their manuscript review, and to Jo-Ann Sire and John Linse for support that went far beyond design and graphics. For living through the research and writing with me, thank you to my daughter Emily Sturdivant and partner Martin Tollefson.

Lastly thank you to Robin Abel who decided I was the person to connect the untold stories of those affected by what happened to Maria on February 22, 2004 with her own journey.

"Have you ever had a rock hit your windshield?
That's how quickly you too could become a victim."

Robin Abel

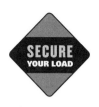

Groups that have invited me to share the story:

King County Traffic Safety
Coalition Group

Foushée & Associates Co.

Fisher and Sons Construction

Governor's Health and Safety
Conference 2005, 2006 and
2007and 2008

Annual Traffic Safety Conf.-
Evergreen Safety Council
2005/2006/2007

Washington Traffic Safety
Commission: Leavenworth 2006

City of Renton

City of Kirkland

City of Bellevue

City of Tacoma

Cannon Construction Inc.

Seattle Public Utilities-North
and South

City of Seattle-North and South
waste facilities

Renton Kiwanis- both afternoon
and morning groups

Waste Management-Seattle,
Auburn, Bremerton, Woodinville,
(6 offices)

Boeing Company

Renton Rotary-lunch group

Sons of Italy-Tacoma

Mowat Construction Company-
both Washington and Oregon
offices

Robin Smith-Bellingham

Labor and Industries in Tukwila

King County Department of
Transportation, Road Services
Division (4 visits)

Pierce County Road Crew

Wilder Construction

Keithly Electric Co.

Puget Sound Safety Group

Educational video with producer

King County Parks

King County "Secure Your Load"
Campaign Kick-Off Media Event at
Qwest Field

Associated General Constructors
Safety Committee

Brian Cyers: group of property
managers

Luke Esser's re-election breakfast

King County Solid Waste
"scale operators"

Washington State Ferry Safety Board

Senate and House Committees (4)

Chelan Public Utility District
-Wenatchee

Highline Community College-
Law Class

Lydig Construction

Bates Technical College-
WSP and Truckers

PCL Civil Southeast-Central Link
Light Rail

Washington State Patrol-Pierce
County Commercial Division

City of Kent-Maintenance Division

"I can't tell you how to secure your load, all I can say is secure your load as if everyone you love is driving in the car behind you."

Robin Abel

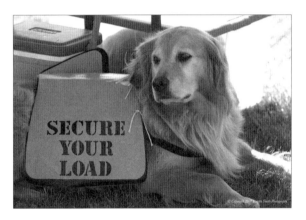

Sky in Wenatchee at Chelan Public Utility event
Photo courtesy of Lynnette Smith Photography LLC

For tips on securing your load and more information please visit the Department of Ecology at www.ecy.wa.gov/programs/swfa/litter.

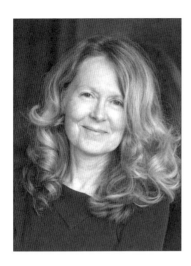

Robin Abel is a Northwest native whose life was altered by the incident that nearly killed her daughter Maria Federici. She would prefer to live a quiet life with her golden retrievers and garden but is compelled to share this story in order to prevent future tragedies due to unsecured loads.